You and Your Cardiologist

A CLEVELAND CLINIC GUIDE

Curtis Mark Rimmerman, M.D.

Cleveland Clinic Press
Cleveland, Ohio

You and Your Cardiologist

A CLEVELAND CLINIC GUIDE

Cleveland Clinic Press • All rights reserved
Copyright © 2008 Cleveland Clinic

Contact:
Cleveland Clinic Press
9500 Euclid Avenue NA32 / Cleveland, Ohio 44195
216-445-5547 / delongk@ccf.org
www.clevelandclinicpress.org

This book is not intended to replace personal medical care and supervision. There is no substitute for the experience and information that your doctor can provide. Rather, it is our hope that this book will provide additional information that will help people understand the nature and delivery of cardiovascular medicine.

Proper medical care always should be tailored to the individual patient. If you read something in this book that seems to conflict with your doctor's instructions, contact your doctor. Since each case is different, there may be good reasons for individual treatment to differ from the information presented in this book. If you have any questions about any treatment in this book, consult your doctor.

The patient names and cases used in this book are composite cases drawn from several sources.

Library of Congress Cataloging-in-Publication Data

Rimmerman, Curtis M.
You and your cardiologist : a Cleveland Clinic guide / Curtis Mark Rimmerman.
p. cm.
ISBN 978-1-59624-081-0 (alk. paper)

1. Heart – Diseases – Popular works. 2. Cardiology – Popular works.
3. Patient education. I. Title.
RC672.R52 2007   616.1'2 – dc22   2007040546

Cover and book design: J. Michael Myers
Medical illustrations: Joe Pangrace, Jeff Loerch; Cleveland Clinic Center for Medical Art and Photography
Photography: Don Gerda, Cleveland Clinic Center for Medical Art and Photography

CONTENTS

Acknowledgments

I would like to thank the thousands of patients I've known through the years. I learn from you every day, and I am privileged to participate with you in improving and maintaining your health.

I would also like to thank Jean Rothman for her expert editorial advice, along with my Cleveland Clinic colleagues, Kathryn DeLong and John Clough, M.D., at Cleveland Clinic Press.

Finally, I would like to thank my wife, Maria, and my daughter, Eleanor, whose continuing encouragement and support are truly immeasurable.

Foreword

The era of paternalistic medicine is over. For my parents'
generation, the advice of their doctor was sacrosanct. Questioning
your physician about diagnostic or treatment options, requesting a
second opinion, or researching to learn more about your disease
just wasn't considered an option. But with the advent of the era of
mass communication, first through cable television, more recently
through the Internet, everything has changed. The amount of
information available to the consumer about health care has
exploded. The increasing knowledge and transparency have
improved medicine, but this change in culture has created a new
problem: information overload. If you conduct a "Google search"
for the term "mitral valve prolapse," you get 350,000 "hits." So how
do thoughtful patients and their families sort through the available
information?

Dr. Curtis Rimmerman, in this book, has made it easy. In a
succinct and readable text, Dr. Rimmerman has synthesized a huge
amount of useful advice. His approach goes beyond the usual
medical book for lay readers. Like other authors, he informs the
thoughtful patient about what one must know about cardiovascular
diseases, diagnostic tests, and therapeutic options. However, Dr.
Rimmerman also provides practical advice on how to get the most
value from the encounter with the cardiovascular practitioner.
Both patients and their physicians will benefit from his advice.
A well-prepared patient leaves the doctor's office with much more

of the knowledge that counts and gains insights that have great long-term value. The physician also benefits because the patient encounter is always more satisfying when the patient provides clear and accurate information. Dr. Rimmerman's insights into becoming a well-prepared patient are unique and refreshing.

Heart disease is one of those conditions that stimulate great fear and anxiety in patients and their families. The antidote to fear is knowledge. Dr. Rimmerman doesn't minimize the seriousness of this illness; rather, he calmly outlines the information patients need to overcome the fear and uncertainty that accompany a diagnosis of heart disease. This book is essential reading for any patient with cardiovascular disease. Dr. Rimmerman's simple and common-sense explanations elegantly inform the reader about essential facts and convey practical advice. It's a great alternative to sorting through 350,000 Google "hits."

Steven E. Nissen, M.D.
Chairman, Department of Cardiovascular Medicine
Cleveland Clinic

Introduction

About This Book

An appointment with a new physician, let alone a cardiologist, can easily generate fear and anxiety. Your mind runs rampant: Heart attack, open-heart surgery, and even death loom large.

This book is meant to reduce those fears. Its purpose is to allow you to step back from the apprehension and take some positive action. It provides you with all the information you need to maximize your relationship with your cardiologist – which can be a great boon to your optimal cardiac health.

As with any life challenge, preparation increases the odds of a successful outcome, so preparing properly for your cardiology appointments is important.

In many ways, planning for your appointment helps level the playing field, permitting you to provide more information to your cardiologist and setting the stage for a more in-depth discussion of your diagnosis and treatment options.

By carefully reading this book, taking notes along the way, and developing your personalized appointment game plan, you will have a full working knowledge of your current and past health. Sharing this with your cardiologist increases the probability that you will get an accurate diagnosis and the best possible treatment. Ultimately that should mean less testing, fewer medications, fewer invasive and uncomfortable procedures, and years added to your life!

HOW TO USE THIS BOOK

The concept for this book grew out of my 14 years as a practicing cardiologist at Cleveland Clinic in Cleveland, Ohio. On a daily basis, I have seen – and continue to see – patients who arrive woefully underprepared for their appointments.

A simple question such as "Why are you here?" can result in a paralyzing silence in the examination room while the patient searches for the right words. Past surgeries and their dates are difficult to recollect with 100 percent accuracy. Essential procedures and relevant past testing often are omitted. And it is rare for a patient to arrive with a full list of accurate medications and dosages, a critical component of any medical discussion.

Unfortunately, a physician has only a finite amount of time to spend with each patient. Doctors often have schedules that are crammed with more patients to see, numerous phone calls and e-mails to answer, and time-consuming hospital rounds to conduct.

If most of your appointment time is spent on information transfer, little time is left for the physical examination and planning of the right diagnostic testing and treatment. Your preparation for your visit will streamline it and place you in the highest tier of patients – those who arrive at their appointment having contemplated their personal health history and prepared it in advance. Perhaps I haven't convinced you yet that this is important, or maybe it sounds like too much work, but I can assure you that it yields huge advantages to your health.

It's best to read the chapters of this book in the order that they are presented. They begin with the assumption that your knowledge of cardiovascular medicine is not extensive. From there, each chapter builds on understandings developed in the previous chapters.

WHAT YOU'LL DISCOVER

I have made every effort to address the complexities of cardiovascular medicine in an understandable and clear format. I will introduce you to the world of cardiology and its subspecialty areas and arm you with critical information to use as you choose a cardiologist. I describe in depth how to make the most of your important first meeting with your cardiologist, reviewing what will happen, outlining how to prepare, and analyzing and detailing each component of your encounter.

Following this, I explain many of the more common cardiac tests, diagnoses, and medicines. It's important for you to know the variety of tests available, what your diagnosis means, and the many kinds of cardiac medications available. This information will make it easier for you to understand your physical condition and help you formulate questions for your doctor before you undergo testing and treatment.

Progressing through the book, you will feel your confidence increase as your fear and anxiety about your cardiology appointments transform into self-assurance and empowerment.

I have included real-life case histories. You will note that each patient responds to his or her illness differently. This is an important point to remember. If you suffer from heart disease, it's likely you know other people who do, too – loved ones, friends, colleagues, relatives. But you won't all react in the same way. I can guarantee it.

If you use the ideas described in this book, you will be well on the way to an excellent relationship with your cardiologist that could significantly benefit your health and well-being in the years to come.

With best wishes for your continued cardiac health,
Curtis Mark Rimmerman, M.D.

Chapter 1

That First Meeting

ROBERT'S MIND IS RACING

Robert glances at the digital clock on his car dashboard – 12:08 p.m. – and then to Carlene, his wife of 36 years, who shifts anxiously in the passenger's seat. I'm 58, he thinks to himself. *I'm too young to be doing this.*

Robert's eyes return to the road in front of him, but his mind is like a rear-view mirror, focusing on alarming images from the past two weeks. One minute, he's jogging on the treadmill at the local YMCA, thinking of ways to shave some strokes off his golf score. The next minute, he's staring wide-eyed at himself in one of the gym's mirrors, holding his hand over his heart and feeling slight pain in his chest. *This isn't good*, he recalls thinking. *My heart is beating way too fast. What's going on? Okay, this hurts, but I'm not hunched over or writhing on the floor. This isn't a heart attack or a stroke. What in the world is it?*

"I went too fast on the treadmill," he told Carlene after driving home from the YMCA. "Also, I drank three cups of coffee before working out. I usually have just one. Maybe the problem is too much caffeine. I'll cut back."

But the accelerated heartbeat happened again, two days later, while Robert was watching his beloved Cleveland Indians play an afternoon baseball game on TV. The *thump thump thump* was rapid and took him by surprise. He wasn't exercising; he was just *sitting there.* He remembers looking down at his chest and thinking of the word "jittery." The episode lasted about 20 minutes. He was relieved when it passed.

"Well, the Indians will do that to anyone," Robert joked to his wife later at the dinner table. "True fans *should* have a heart condition until the team finds a power-hitting third baseman who doesn't boot groundballs."

But he knew something was wrong. Carlene did, too. At bedtime that night she looked into his face and saw fear. That's when he turned to her and said, "I know, I know … I should get this checked out."

So here they are, driving to meet with a cardiologist for the first time. The dashboard clock now reads 12:11 p.m. – 49 minutes before Robert's scheduled appointment. What will that be like? He doesn't feel jittery now, just *nervous.* So nervous he couldn't eat lunch.

His stomach feels like a soup of emotions. One ingredient is fear. Robert pictures himself lying on a hospital bed with an IV in his arm, his three worried children around him. His own dad had died in his early 60s of a heart attack.

Another ingredient is frustration. Robert had just retired and started working out routinely, mostly jogging or brisk walking. A visit with a cardiologist is his reward? People should have seen him in his teens, when he was slim and a star athlete in high school!

Yet another ingredient is guilt. For years Robert had worked as a public school teacher and assistant principal, refusing to rest on weekends – or on his laurels. He was wildly successful, but frequently stressed. On some days, the strain was downright palpable. Maybe he should have tried to relax more often. And maybe he should have watched his weight; he had gained something like an extra 30 pounds over the years.

Robert points to the medical office ahead, and Carlene looks at his hands. She sees lines of sweat. A few minutes later, at 12:21, Robert parks the car and walks hand in hand with his wife toward the entrance to the building.

It's almost time for Robert and Carlene to meet the cardiologist. Their minds seem to be racing even faster than Robert's heart.

DR. SMITH IS RACING, TOO

Dr. John Smith isn't there yet. He's racing against his own schedule – an extensive to-do list that would make most people's heads spin. He's leaving the hospital, 30 minutes from his office, eager to begin his afternoon outpatient clinic. Like Robert, he won't eat lunch today.

Dr. Smith's first afternoon appointment is Robert, scheduled for 1 p.m. He's supposed to see eight patients this afternoon, three of whom (Robert included) are new ones who need comprehensive physical exams and require more time than returning patients.

This morning at the hospital, several incidents had delayed Dr. Smith's office arrival. He examined his 10 hospitalized patients, assessing their medical progress and reviewing test results; in addition, several patients arrived unexpectedly at the emergency room with acute medical problems.

On the drive from the hospital to his office, Dr. Smith contemplated how to recoup his lost time and still deliver attentive care without his patients incurring significant appointment delays.

He is highly regarded by colleagues and patients alike, a man who publishes in respected medical journals and, more important, takes time to understand his patients' fears and personalities. He realizes that he needs to return to the hospital later today to follow up on additional test results for his hospitalized patients. As he glances at his watch, he hopes that his patients have prepared for their visits. On days like this, advance preparation on the part of his patients pays big dividends. It saves a lot of time and actually lets Dr. Smith focus more closely on diagnostic planning.

FIRST-VISIT CONSIDERATIONS

For a patient, a visit to a physician's office often can be filled with apprehension. Meeting the physician for the first time generates unease and a prevailing sense of pressure to provide important, detailed information within a limited span of time.

It isn't easy, especially because patients are often preoccupied with thoughts about their health ("I don't want to die"), loved ones ("I don't want my family to see me like this"), or circumstances ("I need to get better and back on the job ASAP") instead of what the physician actually says.

When patients are distracted like this, it has a direct impact on how much information they retain after the appointment. Their anxiety can impede accurate follow-though, which may include their taking medications correctly, pursuing recommended lifestyle changes, and undergoing future medical testing.

When you're visiting a cardiologist for the first time, you're literally talking about matters of the heart. The whole idea can seem daunting. Concerns abound regarding possible diagnoses, examination findings, diagnostic testing, and treatment implications. And that's *after* you arrive at your appointment: The first visit often requires navigating to an unfamiliar location – perhaps to a large medical center with a confusing array of buildings, signs, and parking options.

Accumulated stress can erode the purpose of evaluating your health concerns. That purpose entails improving the quality of your life and making sure that nothing serious underlies your symptoms.

For these reasons, preparing for your visit ahead of time is extremely valuable. It can mean the difference between your leaving the doctor's office with a less than optimal understanding of your diagnosis and only a foggy notion of what to do next, or feeling well informed, upbeat, and knowledgeable about your next steps.

ADVANCE PREPARATION IS KEY

How do you derive maximum benefit from your appointment with your cardiologist? In light of the demands on your physician's time (a full schedule of outpatients and hospitalized patients, the need to be available in emergencies, and perhaps teaching duties at a medical school), your advance preparation, undertaken days, weeks, and even years before the appointment, can make a great difference. In a word, it can be lifesaving.

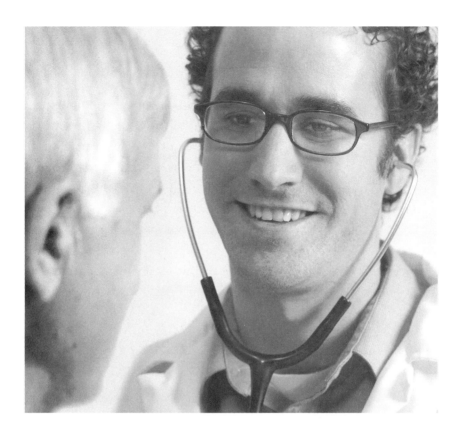

This preparation is crucial, as a successful doctor's visit requires accurate, succinct accounting of your current medical problem coupled with a precise recounting of your medical and surgical history. Doctors refer to this as "presenting."

A successful visit with a physician requires more than a physical exam and a therapeutic medical plan. It requires an accurate *exchange of information,* including both your historical details and the specifics about your current problem. With this type of information exchange, your cardiologist has the best possible vantage point from which to diagnose and treat you.

> The key to maximizing your meeting is simple – advance preparation and organization. When patients arrive prepared and organized, physicians can get to the "heart of the matter" more quickly and effectively. The result is simple and deserved: Quality time that leads to improved health.

WHAT YOU NEED TO KNOW

Current Details

The details of your current problem are usually easier to know than those of past problems, but they're often difficult to describe. What are your symptoms? Which ones are dominant? If you feel pain, what *kind* of pain do you feel and *where?* Exactly *how long* have you felt like this? Pinpointing these and other facts requires thought. Succinctly accounting for a presenting medical problem most often requires a period of self-reflection, best done away from the pressurized setting of a physician's office. This may take the form of a handwritten note, a typewritten summary, or a description to a family member or friend who organizes the information and prepares it for the physician in advance.

Historical Information

As a physician, I believe it's essential for patients to construct a detailed health file for each family member, starting when each is young and continuing with updates as medical events transpire. The process of gathering historical information should not be rushed or driven by an acute medical problem. Instead, it should be a *lifelong endeavor.* By no means should your record be confined to cardiac issues. It will help no matter what health problem might show up.

This strategy may take the form of file folders arranged annually, every five years, or even by decades if most health visits are preventive. When medical encounters and procedures become more frequent, organization by dates with associated brief narratives can help.

A computerized format provides you with easy access, long-term storage, and the ability to update quickly. If you own a scanner, important official test results can be scanned and downloaded into your health record. Just be sure to back up your documents as you would do with all computer data. If you don't use a computer, don't worry – handwritten notes are just fine.

No matter the format of your medical file, having a detailed, chronological record of your health history is critical. (We'll get into more detail in Chapter 4.)

THE BENEFIT OF HAVING SUPPORT

Often, a trusted family member or friend will accompany the patient into the exam room for the physician visit. This often provides a calming influence as the patient isn't proceeding through the appointment process and examination alone.

This support person can serve as a vital set of "extra eyes and ears," listening intently as the physician explains his findings and recommendations. This person also can record information, taking notes that can be reviewed after the visit.

In my experience, the friend or relative accompanying the patient often asks at least one additional insightful question or provides supplemental historical or observational details that are of great help.

For example, consider this patient-care scenario I experienced recently. A woman was referred to me by her primary care physician for evaluation of chest discomfort. Her background included a number of medical problems, including a previous stroke, and it was difficult for her to recall her historical medical details precisely.

The woman was accompanied by her daughter, who provided most of the information. After asking a series of questions, I was able to have the patient describe to the best of her ability the character, severity, and location of her chest discomfort, what precipitated it, and what exacerbated it. In fact, it had been present for years, often occurring at rest and with no clear relationship to her activity level. She had undergone many stress tests in the past, each returning normal and not conclusively supporting coronary artery obstruction.

After our long exchange of information, including a physical examination, I told her my recommendations, which included a coronary angiogram (cardiac catheterization). The patient readily agreed as she wanted to know with certainty whether she had a blockage.

WHAT IS A CORONARY ANGIOGRAM?

A coronary angiogram, also known as a cardiac catheterization, is performed to detect the presence and assess the severity of any coronary artery blockages. It involves the introduction of a catheter (a long tube approximately the diameter of a piece of cooked spaghetti) into the blood vessels through a small entry point in the groin. The catheter is advanced until it reaches the coronary ostia – the openings of your left and right coronary arteries. There, "contrast agent" (dye) is carefully injected into the artery, opacifying and therefore creating an arterial image on special, simultaneously obtained x-rays. If there are any blockages, they should show up on the x-rays.

For a more complete description of coronary angiography, see Chapter 5.

Just before I was about to leave the exam room, the patient's daughter added that she thought she remembered her mother undergoing a heart catheterization at a local hospital approximately nine months earlier, and she thought the results had been normal.

By means of a quick phone call, within five minutes I had arranged for the results to be faxed to my office. Seeing that the results were indeed normal, I confidently canceled the heart catheterization. The likelihood that a severe narrowing of the coronary artery had developed over the previous nine months was exceedingly low.

Thanks to the astute recollection of her daughter, the patient was able to avoid an invasive procedure that would have required mild sedation and a lost day of work. In addition, although cardiac catheterization is very safe, there is a small risk of a complication such as bleeding, clotting, damage to blood vessels, or infection at the site where the catheter is introduced – all of which the patient avoided.

Later, it was confirmed that the woman was suffering from musculoskeletal discomfort of the chest wall. I prescribed over-the-counter medications and her symptoms improved.

Guidelines for Supporters

If a family member or friend accompanies you for a physician appointment, everyone should observe guidelines to maximize the value of the time-limited interaction. It should be a priority to allocate time for a direct verbal exchange between the physician and the patient. This interaction must maintain precedence. Only the patient can communicate to the physician exactly what symptoms he or she is experiencing.

The supporter shouldn't disrupt the detailed one-on-one interaction between the patient and the physician. Instead, the family member or friend is encouraged to wait for a quiet moment and then provide supplemental information concerning the patient's medical history, accurately and concisely providing historical details. The supporter also can provide valuable observational data for the physician, such as "He is now more short of breath ascending stairs, his appetite is less, and he is taking more nitroglycerin tablets."

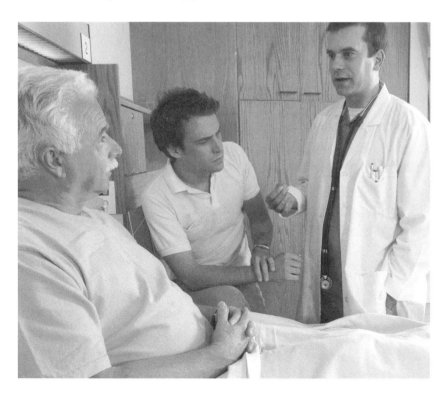

CHARACTERIZING YOUR SYMPTOMS

What does it mean when the doctor asks about the character of your pain? Well, pain can be characterized or described in many ways, and some of those ways hold important clues for an accurate diagnosis. A cardiologist may listen for such key words as "squeezing," "heavy," "sharp," "dull," "like a knife," "like a lightning bolt." By providing as much information as possible, descriptions like these help him evaluate your situation.

The supporter can also relay symptoms and feelings the patient may have mentioned in the past but doesn't presently recall.

When he receives such historical information in an organized, typewritten format, the physician is able to focus even more intently on the patient's current presenting concern, reducing the need for detailed questioning of past medical conditions.

If at all possible, it's also smart for the patient and supporter to rehearse before the visit. (The supporter takes the role of the cardiologist.) This will help the patient focus on current symptoms and think ahead of time how to best communicate them in a cogent manner.

These steps save time for everyone, allowing the physician to focus on the salient facts without delay, with plenty of time for follow-up questions.

INTERACTING WITH A SPECIALIST

Unlike a primary care physician, a specialist focuses on a narrower aspect of your health. For example, a gastroenterologist focuses on diseases of the digestive tract, a neurologist on conditions affecting the nervous system.

In many respects, a specialist possesses an advantage over a primary care physician because he can concentrate his attention primarily on one organ system. You, the patient, also possess an advantage because you are able to prepare for the specialist's more focused approach.

When organizing information for your cardiology appointment, you can focus on your cardiac concerns more than on other health problems. You can prioritize your medical and surgical histories, listing those items first that have a higher likelihood of contributing to a cardiac symptom. (An example of a patient's detailed medical history is included in Chapter 3.)

Many of us have long medical histories, but a cardiologist will be most concerned about issues affecting your visit to him – the factors that pertain to his specialization. For example:

- Are you a longstanding diabetic?
- What are your tobacco habits?
- Do your first-degree relatives have a history of premature coronary artery disease?
- What's your average blood pressure and what have your past blood cholesterol and triglyceride levels been?

These pieces of information are more relevant and helpful than, for example, knowledge about the removal of a benign mole or treatment of a broken leg.

Why You Want to Avoid Extraneous Information

It's not possible for a specialist (or for that matter, any physician) to evaluate and develop a treatment plan addressing a range of concerns in a single visit. Presenting an extensive list of discussion points will make for an inefficient visit. Instead, develop realistic expectations of your appointment goals before meeting the physician.

Consider ranking your symptoms and concerns, and commit to communicating and focusing on the five most important. Should the cardiologist ask further questions, it may be entirely appropriate to move down your list and include more information. Just keep in mind that within the time limits of the appointment, it's extremely difficult to give adequate consideration to a series of different complaints, especially those outside the scope of the specialist's practice.

By coupling your process of self-education with careful preparation, you can "steer" your cardiology appointment to maximize the exchange of relevant data. The result will be a successful appointment that leads to your better health.

HOW IS ROBERT?

As for Robert, his story has a happy ending, but I won't reveal it just yet. We'll be keeping track of his progress throughout the book as he is diagnosed, tested, and treated. ◆

Chapter 2

Choosing a Cardiologist

Your primary care physician has told you that you need to see a cardiologist. Before you choose one, you should know as much as possible about your choices and about the world of cardiology. In fact, by beginning to seek this information, you've taken your first steps on the road to a successful relationship with your cardiologist.

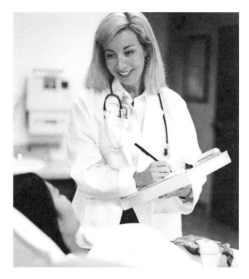

Let's start with a basic question: What does a cardiologist do? Ask virtually anyone, and the most common answer will probably be "treats heart problems." More technically, a cardiologist is a physician specializing in the evaluation and treatment of heart and blood-vessel disorders.

But cardiologists are concerned with much more than heart attacks, congestive heart failure, stroke, or other cardiac-related disorders. Most also see patients whose cardiovascular conditions are caused by or associated with out-of-control diabetes, high blood pressure, congenital disorders, peripheral artery disease, tobacco use, or high cholesterol, all of which also need to be evaluated and treated.

Better yet, those conditions can be *prevented*, and this is also the realm of the cardiologist. Cardiologists create a program that enables patients to live healthier lives both before and after a problem is diagnosed and treated.

A HUGE – AND GROWING – PROBLEM

Heart disease, despite new medications and successful surgical interventions, is still the leading killer in the United States – for both men and women. According to the Centers for Disease Control and Prevention, cardiovascular disease causes about one death every minute among women, claiming nearly half a million female lives each year. That's more lives than the next seven causes of death *combined.*

Heart disease is more deadly than all other modern scourges, including cancer and loss of life from car accidents, crimes, and war. (Cancer is next, at about 20 percent of all deaths.)

Contrary to popular assumption, adults aren't the only group at risk. Cardiovascular disease ranks as the No. 3 cause of death (behind conditions originating in the perinatal period and accidents) for children younger than age 15, according to the CDC.

In the next 12 months, about 25,000 babies will be born with congenital heart defects. About a fourth of this number will die, and the survivors will join the nearly half-million people who are living with heart defects.

HEART PROBLEMS BY THE NUMBERS

79,400,000 million	People in the United States suffering from some form of heart disease in 2004
1 out of every 2.8	Number of deaths from cardiovascular disease
33	Seconds between each death from cardiovascular disease
$403.1 billion	Cost of cardiovascular disease and stroke in 2006 according to the American Heart Association and the National Heart, Lung, and Blood Institute.

A Long Training Period

The road to becoming a cardiologist requires discipline, focus, and perseverance. Your cardiologist has devoted years to studying general internal medicine and three more years at least simply to earn recognition as a board-certified specialist in cardiovascular disease.

It's common for cardiologists to spend additional years training in a specific field such as interventional cardiology (becoming experts in procedures such as angioplasty and stenting) or nuclear cardiology (developing expertise in the diagnosis and visualization of heart blockages). Other areas of specialty include echocardiography (recording and interpreting images of the heart) and electrophysiology (working with the heart's electrical function).

Beyond all this education, your cardiologist may choose to specialize even further by focusing on specific patient groups such as children or very elderly people.

This is clearly a long path to take. So what's the lure? It's quite simple: Cardiovascular disease is the leading cause of death in the Western world and represents a huge opportunity to make a positive impact on public health.

THE FOUR MAIN SUBSPECIALTIES

The number and type of cardiac disorders are vast, but they can be broken down into four main categories:

- Plumbing (blood vessels)
- Electrical (rhythm disorders)
- Muscular (congestive heart failure)
- Valves (leaks and restricted openings)

These disorders often overlap, complicating evaluation and treatment. For example, if a person with a blocked coronary artery suffers a heart attack, the weakening of the heart muscle may lead to fluid retention. It may also cause incomplete valve closure, resulting in significant valve leakage that then leads to serious heart-rhythm disturbances.

Let's briefly look at each of the four types of cardiac disorders.

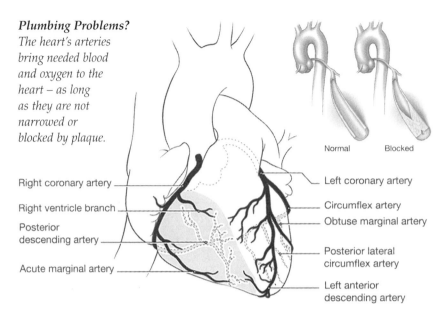

Plumbing Problems?
The heart's arteries
bring needed blood
and oxygen to the
heart – as long
as they are not
narrowed or
blocked by plaque.

Normal   Blocked

Right coronary artery

Right ventricle branch

Posterior
descending artery

Acute marginal artery

Left coronary artery

Circumflex artery

Obtuse marginal artery

Posterior lateral
circumflex artery

Left anterior
descending artery

"Plumbing"

Just like the rest of the body, the heart needs a plentiful supply of oxy-gen-rich blood to operate properly. The blood is brought to the heart through arteries. (See illustration above.) For the purposes of our analogy, think of these arteries as pipes.

Just as water cannot flow through a clog in your sink pipe at home, if one of the heart's "pipes" is narrowed or blocked, the fresh oxygen-rich blood can't flow properly to the heart. Blockages that clog a coronary artery are composed of plaque, which includes a variety of blood prod-ucts and fatty substances, including cholesterol.

This "plumbing problem" can result in chest pain as blood supply is slowed by the narrowing of the artery and, if left untreated, heart attack.

"Electrical"

The human body includes a delicate network of electrical fibers. In the heart, they are concentrated in anatomically specialized "pacemaker" areas where they branch or "arborize" like a tree to serve the entire heart muscle.

The electrical signals generated in the heart govern the rate and rhythm of the heartbeat by controlling the contraction and relaxation of the heart's four chambers (two upper chambers, called atria, and two lower chambers, called ventricles).

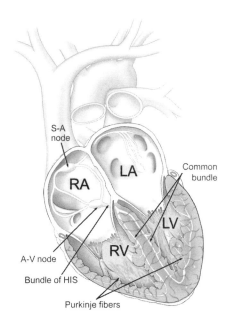

Under normal conditions, the cardiac electrical impulse is transmitted in fractions of a second, resulting in simultaneous coordinated contractions of the heart chambers at a regular pace. But in abnormal situations, the electrical signals can cause the heart to beat in an uncoordinated fashion, resulting in heartbeats that are too fast, too slow, and even chaotic.

Rhythm disorders encompass the full spectrum of severity. They can be "innocent" (an occasional premature heartbeat) or life-threatening (heartbeats that are fast and unstable).

If you have an electrical-system abnormality, you may feel your heart racing or notice palpitations. These symptoms may be coupled with lightheadedness, near-fainting, or passing out.

ROBERT'S "ELECTRICAL" PROBLEM

If you guessed that Robert could be suffering from a problem in his heart's electrical system, you're correct. He feels his heart beating too fast, even when he's just sitting in front of the television.

Although Robert will need further testing, Dr. Smith suspects an atrial rhythm abnormality, an irregular heart rhythm emanating from his upper cardiac chambers. An atrial rhythm abnormality occurs when the electrical signals fire too rapidly, causing the muscles in the atria to contract too quickly. This leads to the kind of fast heartbeat Robert is experiencing.

Heart-rhythm disturbances are often associated with (but not limited to) previous heart damage and muscle weakening.

Cardiology specialists who treat the most complex heart-rhythm disturbances are called electrophysiologists.

"Muscular"

Much of the heart is composed of a unique form of muscle tissue called cardiac muscle, or myocardium. ("Myo" denotes muscle and "cardium" denotes heart.) Heart-muscle abnormalities take two forms:

- Weakened and thinned muscle
- Strong and thickened muscle

Weakened and thinned heart muscle can't pump blood out of the heart to the body as well as normal heart muscle can. This abnormality may result from damage caused by a heart attack or the effect of a previous virus on the heart.

Also, longstanding untreated valvular heart disease can overwork and fatigue the heart muscle, rendering it irreversibly weakened.

Patients with a weakened heart muscle are prone to developing congestive heart failure (CHF), in which the heart cannot pump enough blood to the body. CHF can result in fluid retention, breathlessness, kidney dysfunction, and premature death.

Another form of congestive heart failure that is being increasingly recognized in the medical community is "diastolic" heart failure, which is a failure of the heart muscle to relax. Diastolic heart failure most often occurs in patients who have poorly controlled high blood pressure and abnormally thickened heart muscle. In circumstances such as this, the heart muscle is strong, but pressures in the heart are elevated, causing blood to engorge the lungs.

"Valves"

Four heart valves reside within the heart, each integral to the proper directional flow of blood. In normal situations, the valves serve as one-way gates, directing blood in an unimpeded forward direction and preventing blood backflow.

When a heart valve is diseased, it either doesn't open or doesn't close properly. In either case, this places undue stress on the heart muscle, rendering it susceptible to fatigue and weakening.

Valve abnormalities, depending on their extent, reduce heart-pumping efficiency. In advanced situations, cardiac valve abnormalities are best addressed with surgical repair or replacement.

HOW TO CHOOSE A CARDIOLOGIST

No matter whether the problem is in the plumbing, electrical system, muscles, or valves, choosing the right cardiologist is one of the most important life decisions that you can make.

Most often, your primary care doctor can provide expert guidance when you're looking for the specialist in the community – or further afield – who may be the best suited to handle your needs.

The old cliché "it takes two to tango" perfectly describes how the ideal patient/cardiologist relationship would ultimately function. Each of you will have certain expectations of one another and certain contributions you can make to ensure that the professional relationship is a strong one.

Let's start with your expectations.

For the moment, let's assume that your first meeting with your cardiologist won't be the result of an urgent trip to the emergency room. So either your primary care physician referred you or you referred yourself (this is known as a "self-referral"). You are most likely to meet your cardiologist at her office.

Different heart abnormalities may require different specialists. For example, if a "plumbing" problem is under consideration, a cardiologist specializing in cardiac catheterization, angioplasty, and stenting may be best. Heart-rhythm disorders are evaluated and treated most effectively by specialists known as electrophysiologists. Certain physicians, particularly in large medical centers, specialize in heart-valve abnormalities while others are experts in treating congestive heart failure.

You'll want to find out what sort of training your cardiologist has completed. (See "Resources for Finding a Cardiologist," page 20.)

Next, check out the doctor's credentials. The first place to go is your hospital's Office of Medical Staff Affairs (names for this office may vary a bit from hospital to hospital). Here, you should be able to obtain a list of cardiologists who have admitting privileges to the hospital, how long they've been on staff, and their specialty interests within cardiology.

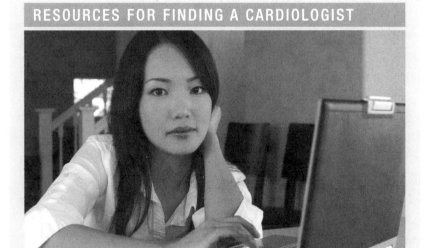

RESOURCES FOR FINDING A CARDIOLOGIST

When you're looking for a doctor, your state medical board is a good resource. While each state is governed by its own board, every state keeps information on each practitioner's date of birth, office address, areas of specialization, and – most important – history of disciplinary action.

Most state medical boards have websites where you can gain access to this information. Also, many physician practices have their own websites where you can search for anything relevant about the doctor. For example, does the doctor have office hours that meet your schedule? At what hospitals does she have staff privileges?

In addition, you can visit the website of the American Board of Internal Medicine (www.abim.org), where you can research each physician's board certification and recertification status.

When you have selected several names, gather as much information as possible about your choices by talking to family members, friends, or co-workers. These kinds of sources should help you learn about each doctor's personality and bedside manner.

What to Ask

Here are some good questions to ask:

1. Is the cardiologist a good communicator? Did she thoroughly explain her findings, testing rationale, and testing results in an understandable manner?

2. Is she responsive? When you called and left a message for her, did she return the call promptly and in a concerned fashion?

3. Was she willing to send your test results to you with an accompanying letter of explanation?

4. How easy was it to schedule an appointment? Was she in high demand? Will you have to wait months for a new-patient appointment?

5. Once you're established as a patient, will it be easy to obtain follow-up appointments? Or is her practice so full that you will have a long wait?

6. Are the members of her office staff (including reception and nursing personnel) professional and kind?

Also, consider asking health-care professionals you know whom *they* would go to if they had a heart problem.

TRUST YOURSELF

The most important factor when determining the right cardiologist, however, may be a simple one: How do you feel about the person and her office when you first meet?

Today's medical environment often limits patient-physician interaction during an office visit so your first impression is likely to be of the office staff. As you complete the inevitable personal information and insurance forms, determine your first impression:

- Were you given help promptly when you had questions?
- Is the office calm or chaotic?
- Do you feel as if you're in a professional environment, or do you feel ignored?
- When the nurse or physician's assistant calls you into the examining room, how is the encounter?

While your doctor's nurse takes some preliminary history and checks your vital signs, you should begin to develop an impression of the doctor's practice. Do you feel comfortable? Have personnel really listened to you, or have they simply taken notes without glancing up or asking you a single personal question beyond the list on the chart?

If something doesn't feel right, make a mental note of it. After your appointment, if you still feel an overall sense of discomfort, you may want to consider trying a different doctor. This may seem bothersome in terms of time and effort, but your relationship with your cardiologist is likely to last a long time. You deserve to find a doctor and a practice where you feel welcomed as a valued participant in your own cardiac care. ◆

Chapter 3

Maximizing Your Appointment Time

PATIENTS AND DOCTORS BOTH WANT QUALITY TIME

Meeting with your physician should be a detailed, interactive experience. You want an optimal encounter that's valuable and efficient, and so does your physician. You deserve to leave his office armed with more knowledge and understanding about your condition and a clear idea of what's coming next.

To that end, as we've said, you should arrive at his office armed with information – about your present illness, your medical history, and other details.

RAY'S STORY

When I think about the importance and benefits of patient preparation, I think of Ray. I met Ray 13 years ago. At the time, he was in his late 50s and ran a highly successful consulting practice. He also was a part-time college lecturer at Ashland University in Ashland, Ohio. And he was in the final stages of completing his doctorate degree, preparing for an upcoming oral defense of his dissertation.

Ray arrived at Cleveland Clinic by helicopter after suffering a major heart attack in Elkins, West Virginia. His medical condition was initially quite serious. His heart muscle had been severely damaged by the heart attack, and shortly after the heart attack he developed symptoms of congestive heart failure.

Ray's heart muscle was so damaged that it was not able to capably propel his blood forward, and some of the blood pooled (congested) in his lungs. This congestion led to shortness of breath, particularly when he was lying down, which tends to increase lung pressures (so-called pulmonary venous hypertension). The increased lung fluid reduced his ability to acquire more oxygen. He had to sit up to breathe, his breathing was labored, and because he had to stop and catch his breath, he couldn't speak in full sentences.

In addition, when enough blood is not propelled out of the heart, all the body's organs are affected because they're getting less blood than usual.

STARTING OFF ON THE RIGHT FOOT

Many things about Ray impressed me during our initial meeting. First, his confidence was unwavering. He demonstrated steadfast support and concern for his family and how his illness was affecting them. He also meticulously prepared for my arrival on hospital rounds with carefully considered, insightful questions. He clearly articulated how he was feeling physically.

Ray required more time than most patients, but it was time I happily provided. Our close interaction enhanced my understanding of him as well as his understanding of our treatment plan.

Having used this clear information as well as his medical signs and symptoms to diagnose congestive heart failure, I was able to optimize his medical condition with medications, including:

- Beta blockers to reduce the stress and strain on his heart

- ACE inhibitors to lower his blood pressure, dilate his arteries, and reduce the forward resistance to blood flow (thereby reducing the work of the heart)

- Diuretics to reduce the congestion in his heart and lungs, reduce his circulating blood volume, and increase his urine output by increasing the amount of blood going to his kidneys

These medications stabilized his condition and turned him from what is termed "decompensated" to "compensated" heart failure. (Decompensated heart failure refers to a serious, rapid accumulation of fluid in the lungs that causes shortness of breath and fatigue. When medications can compensate for the heart's condition, it is called compensated heart failure.)

It was then time to discover what had caused Ray's heart attack in the first place. We performed a cardiac catheterization, a procedure that involves injecting x-ray dye into the coronary arteries to locate atherosclerotic blockages.

We identified several blockages as well as weakened heart muscle, confirming my clinical suspicion. I shared with Ray my opinion that he needed to have coronary artery bypass graft surgery, also called CABG, pronounced "cabbage."

THINKING FORWARD, ASKING QUESTIONS

Since he was feeling better, Ray was able to give some thought to his situation. He started asking very insightful questions about his upcoming surgery. He wanted to know what it entailed and what he could do to prepare himself both emotionally and physically for the surgery and its aftereffects.

I showed him a spirometer, a plastic pipe into which a patient blows, supporting lung expansion after surgery. Ray's questions spurred us to give him a spirometer *before* the surgery so that he could practice and learn how to use it when he didn't have an incision and pain in his chest. Ray practiced faithfully, becoming quite facile at using the spirometer, which enhanced his recovery when the time came for him to use it postoperatively.

Mindful of upcoming plans he had made with his family, Ray also asked how long he'd have to stay in the hospital after surgery. He also had some questions about when he'd be able to go back to school and continue his Ph.D. studies.

Considering Medications

Ray asked about the different medications he would be on and their potential side effects. Although these were good questions, I wasn't able to answer some of them because it was difficult to predict what medicines he would be on after surgery. But I was able to give him broad answers, and the fact that he was thinking in such crystal-clear terms before the surgery showed me that he was already looking ahead, past his surgical period.

I find that those patients who are planning their futures before a major cardiac procedure are the ones who have better outcomes. In my experience, a positive attitude is tied to an enhanced outcome after heart surgery or any significant procedure.

> I find that those patients who are planning their futures before a major cardiac procedure are the ones who have better outcomes.

I often refer to heart surgery as a "speed bump" in a person's life, meaning that it's something that slows your progress on an otherwise smooth path, but it doesn't necessarily force you to grind to a halt. Ray shared this point of view. He underwent successful coronary artery bypass graft surgery and was discharged from the hospital five days later. His later recovery was similarly uneventful.

Thirteen years later, Ray continues to see me twice a year for regular checkups. At each visit, we review his medications in detail, perform a focused cardiac examination, and make any needed medication adjustments. He faithfully continues a three-day-a-week routine of exercise in an outpatient cardiac rehabilitation program. He has received his Ph.D. and has retired from his consulting practice, devoting more time to reading and traveling, and to his family.

A STANDARD SEQUENCE OF QUESTIONS

Let's take a closer look at the elements of a typical doctor-patient meeting. This knowledge will help you to prepare for your upcoming physician appointment and contribute to a maximal health outcome.

In medical school and residency training, physicians are taught to accumulate patient data consistently and systematically. Typically, physicians obtain this information verbally and in an eight-part sequence. We'll discuss the first – and most critical – two elements here and examine the rest in Chapter 4.

Chief Complaint

The first subject you and your doctor will discuss is your "chief complaint." This includes your reason for making the appointment and a description of what is bothering you. (Even if you tell your story in sweet and even tones, doctors call this the "complaint.")

The chief complaint is a brief description of why you're seeking medical attention. The physician will usually start with an open-ended question such as "Why are you here?" or "What prompted you to make this appointment?" to elicit this important initial information. From here, the physician can quickly raise additional questions whose answers will help him delve more deeply into your health concern.

It is an unfortunate but necessary fact of life that appointment time is finite. Anything you can do in advance to speed the exchange of information during your visit will pay dividends because it will allow the physician more time to ask the insightful questions that home in on what your symptoms might mean and more time for the physical examination. It will also allow more time for discussion of your treatment plan, medications, and any testing that is planned.

Knowing your chief complaint may seem simple – after all, you know why you made your appointment – but it's often easier to know how you feel than it is to state it.

For example, I recently saw a patient named Rick, whose chief complaint was "not feeling well." When I asked why he was seeing me, he reiterated, "I just don't feel well." I followed up, asking him, "What do you mean?" He repeated the same answer.

This is an example of a chief complaint that hasn't been well thought out. It required additional questioning on my part to extract information. Many patients reply with one-word answers, creating a time-intensive process of information transfer. I am happy to spend time with a patient, but I would rather spend it getting through the preliminaries quickly so that there is more time for serious discussion of the condition and possible treatment plan.

Eventually, I was able to put the pieces of Rick's puzzle together. He had been experiencing fatigue, shortness of breath during physical activity, and central chest pressure for the past three months, increasing in both severity and ease of provocation. Getting to the root of his chief complaint took about 10 minutes of valuable appointment time.

Had Rick been able to communicate his chief complaint succinctly, we would have accomplished much more during the visit. Such a summary might have gone: "For the past three months I have been fatigued, short of breath with activity, and have been noticing pressure in my chest when I walk my dog. These symptoms have been getting worse over time."

With the time saved, we could have delved more deeply into eating habits and a weight-loss strategy, and discussed approaches that would help him quit smoking.

An additional, if obvious, time-saver is for patients to arrive on schedule. I always try to stay on time because my patients' time is as valuable as mine. Out of respect for those patients who follow, sometimes it's necessary to reschedule with a patient who arrives late. Or sometimes I'll have to take less than optimal shortcuts during the appointment, recognizing that I don't have all the information at hand. This is unsatisfying to me and to my patients.

For instance, I recently saw a woman who had relocated to Cleveland from Illinois. She clearly had a cardiac history and brought some information with her, but she was not able to communicate her history with succinctness and accuracy. The information that I was given by the outside physician was incomplete.

I wasn't sure why the patient was on specific medications, nor did I know the timing of her last heart catheterization. These facts were of critical importance. Also, there were conflicting data: I had a report from 1998, but the patient told me that she had had a catheterization in 2004, yet that information was not included in her history.

It can be confusing when the patient doesn't bring accurate information, and it can lead the physician down the wrong diagnostic testing path or to a wrong prescription.

Without vital details, I had to put the appointment on hold and told the patient that I would be in touch with her soon.

I went to my office, dictated a letter, and copied my notes to the outside doctor, asking specific questions that the patient had been unable to answer. A week or two passed before I received the doctor's reply. This delayed my evaluation of her condition by several weeks. Fortunately, in this case there were no serious repercussions to the delay that prevented my making an immediate, accurate diagnosis

BE SURE YOU "COMPLAIN" SUCCINCTLY!

Here are a few examples of a concise chief complaint:

- I've had shortness of breath for the past three months.

- For three weeks I've had chest pressure when I exert myself, with a simultaneous pain in my left arm.

- I've noticed central chest pressure that travels to my throat and left shoulder each time I take my dog for a walk. This has been occurring over the past month and has been increasing in both severity and frequency.

- Over the past two weeks, I've noticed an extremely rapid heartbeat occurring out of the blue with lightheadedness and near-fainting.

- I can't breathe the way I used to and I've gained 20 pounds over the past few weeks. My ankles and feet are twice their previous size.

- Over the past year, I've noticed progressive shortness of breath and reduced ability to perform my daily activities such as grocery-shopping and climbing stairs. My waist size has increased by four inches, but I don't think my calories have increased significantly.

and treatment plan, but in other cardiac cases, the delay might have made a significant difference in the patient's health and quality of life.

Before you verbalize your chief concern, carefully consider your symptoms and prioritize them, naming your most serious one first. It's human nature, even for a physician, to grasp and adhere to the first set of spoken words. That's just one more reason why advance preparation and organization are essential. Bombarding your physician with a set of 10 concerns dating back more than 20 years isn't a "chief complaint" and can't be satisfactorily addressed in one visit.

The more meticulous you are, the more precise your physician's follow-up questions can be and the more accurate and timely his diagnosis.

History of Present Illness

The next major factor your doctor will address is the "history of present illness." This category covers any supplementary details of your chief concern.

The history of present illness provides more detailed information regarding the chief complaint. Typical questions may include:

- When did your symptoms begin?
- Where are they located?
- Do they radiate (travel)?
- What makes them better or worse?
- Are they predictable or random in occurrence?
- Have you experienced them previously?
- How would you grade their severity?
- Are they increasing in severity, frequency, or ease of provocation?
- Have you sought medical attention for these symptoms before?
- Do you have an idea what your symptoms represent?

Accurate and thoughtful answers are the key to a successful first meeting. Broad, open-ended questions from your physician are an important component of your visit and should be expected. Your answers afford you the opportunity to "tell your story" about why you've come to see the physician.

This crucial portion of the visit may dictate the success or failure of your joint doctor-patient interaction. A timely yet complete exchange of information requires a knowledgeable and experienced physician and a well-prepared, accurate patient. If the physician overlooks important questions and/or you deliver inaccurate answers, it can delay the identification of a correct diagnosis and subsequent implementation of a successful treatment plan.

As a patient, you can anticipate some of these questions and provide a written description of your signs and symptoms to your physician. Approach your visit as you might treat a trip to buy a car or any other product: Advance preparation yields a more informed experience and a successful outcome. After all, what stakes are higher than your own health?

It's important not to be influenced by the line of questioning. Rather, remain firm and don't feel compelled to answer a question that you consider irrelevant to your situation. Your answers should be genuine. Focus on what you're feeling – don't rush or unintentionally fabricate just to provide an answer.

Here is a hypothetical exchange in which a few open-ended questions by the physician are used to pinpoint the exact nature of the symptoms, their timing, and duration.

Physician: "Mrs. Jones, it is my pleasure to meet you today. I'm Dr. Smith and I'm one of the heart doctors here at Cleveland Clinic. I have some advance knowledge of why you are here. I've reviewed your recent visits with Dr. Rice, one of our excellent primary care providers. But instead of me being biased about the purpose of your visit today, I'd like to hear from you why you were referred."

Mrs. Jones: "I've been having shortness of breath for about two weeks."

Physician: "Have you been able to identify any circumstances when you might experience this shortness of breath?"

Mrs. Jones: "It happens when I go upstairs or walk really fast, as I did last week when it was raining so hard and I had to get from the parking lot to the grocery store."

Physician: "Are you able to expound on that any further?" (This open-ended question is posed so as not to steer Mrs. Jones into a pigeon-holed answer. The physician is trying to get her to volunteer her symptoms instead of the physician asking suggestive questions that she may latch onto.)

Mrs. Jones: "I'm not sure what you mean."

Physician: "Are you experiencing any other symptoms with your shortness of breath?"

Mrs. Jones: "Come to think of it, I do experience some chest discomfort."

Physician: "Oh really? Where is that chest discomfort located?"

Mrs. Jones: (Points to center of her chest.)

Physician: "Can you tell me anything else about that chest discomfort?"

Mrs. Jones: "Actually, I noticed it since the shortness of breath has come on, and it usually occurs at the same time as the shortness of breath."

Physician: "Can you tell me anything else about the chest discomfort?"

Mrs. Jones: "It's not a sharp pain but more of a sensation of pressure or fullness in my chest."

Physician: "Is there anything else you'd like to tell me about the character of the discomfort?"

Mrs. Jones: "That's pretty much it, but I must say now that I think about it that I've noticed it sometimes in my throat and down my left arm."

Physician: "Is there anything else? How about the duration of the discomfort?"

Mrs. Jones: "I'm not really sure how long it lasts."

Physician: "Let me put it this way, Mrs. Jones: Does it last for seconds, minutes, or hours?"

Mrs. Jones: "I'd have to say minutes."

Physician: "Is it, say, more than 10 minutes? More than 15 minutes?"

Mrs. Jones: "Probably in the range of 5 to 10 minutes."

Physician: "What makes it better?"

Mrs. Jones: "If I stop my activity, it makes it better."

Physician: "What makes it worse?"

Mrs. Jones: "If I really push myself, it makes it worse."

Physician: "What happens if you don't stop your activity?"

Mrs. Jones: "I've never tried that because I'm concerned that it will get worse if I continue."

Physician: "Is there anything else you do that makes it better?"

Mrs. Jones: "Not really."

Physician: "Are there any times that you're not experiencing chest discomfort?"

Mrs. Jones: "When I'm at rest I never experience it, and it has never woken me up."

Physician: "Mrs. Jones, if I asked you if you had chest pain, what would your answer be?"

Mrs. Jones: "I don't have any chest pain. It's not pain, it's discomfort."

The open-ended nature of this dialogue allowed the doctor to elicit Mrs. Jones' answers without biasing her in one way or another. This approach usually lets patients be more reflective of their symptoms, which in turn contributes to an accurate diagnosis more than if a patient is led by the doctor's questions.

Remember, you maintain a powerful advantage because only you are experiencing your symptoms. Only you can effectively and accurately communicate what you're feeling. Interpreting your symptoms and translating them into understandable words is paramount. It's your job to reflect upon your symptoms, perhaps discuss them with family and friends before your appointment, and develop the all-important organized initial presentation to your physician.

Despite your best efforts, your physician may deviate from your preparatory thoughts. This is completely satisfactory and expected. Just try to relax, remain honest, and be frank when you don't know the answer. Don't be afraid to offer an answer that in your mind may only tangentially answer the question. You may reveal details that seem unimportant to you but are highly useful to your skilled physician. Your answers may provoke additional thoughts and lines of questioning, raising the likelihood of an accurate diagnosis, a successful treatment plan, and improved health. After all, this is why you sought the physician's help in the first place!

Let's take a look at another example of a physician-patient dialogue that builds upon a chief complaint and establishes the history of the present illness. We'll use the chief complaint of Rick, mentioned earlier: "For the past three months I've been fatigued, short of breath with activity, and have been noticing chest pressure when I walk my dog."

Physician: "What do you mean by *fatigued?*"

Patient: "When I used to walk my dog, I was able to walk for 30 minutes without stopping. Now, I feel short of breath and need to sit down and rest after only 10 minutes."

Physician: "Now, about the fatigue. Are you tired?"

Patient: "No, my muscles and energy level are fine. It's the shortness of breath that limits me."

Physician: "Is this progressing in severity? Is the shortness of breath more easily induced?"

Patient: "Yes to both. I've had to cut back my activities significantly."

Physician: "Tell me about the chest pressure. Where is it located? Does it move or radiate to other areas?"

Patient: "It stays in the middle of my chest. It feels as if there's a ball being squeezed in my chest."

Physician: "Does this occur at rest, when you're active, or both?"

Patient: "It occurs only when I'm really active, but I've been noticing it when I exert myself less as well. It also has been more intense recently."

Physician: "I'm concerned about a heart-artery blockage. Do any close relatives have a history of heart artery blockages, heart attack, balloons, stents, or bypass surgery?"

Patient: "Yes, my father had a bypass operation when he was 49, and his father died from a heart attack. I'm not sure how old he was."

Physician: "How about your cholesterol values and blood pressure?

Patient: "I haven't had my cholesterol checked in a while. My blood pressure is usually 140/80."

Physician: "Do you have a history of smoking?"

Patient: "I used to smoke two packs a day for 20 years. I quit when I started experiencing the shortness of breath and chest discomfort."

This exchange took about two minutes. It was focused and succinct, derived from an extremely well-stated chief complaint. It established the lack of true fatigue, instead identifying central squeezing chest discomfort and shortness of breath upon exertion as the predominant symptoms. The physician learned that both symptoms are intensifying and are more easily induced.

Why was it helpful to elicit these symptom patterns and risk factors from the patient? It led the physician down a more urgent and invasive testing path. The symptom intensification suggested that a noninvasive external evaluation (i.e., stress test) did not make sense. Instead, the changing pattern of chest discomfort and the possible accelerating pattern of cardiac symptoms suggested that a more urgent evaluation in the form of a heart catheterization would be required. Also, the dialogue identified risk factors for coronary artery disease, heightening the level of concern.

Normally, co-existent conditions such as high blood pressure and high cholesterol are best relegated to the medical history section. (See next chapter.) But when the history of present illness is focused upon the possibility of obstructive coronary artery disease, the doctor may selectively "import" components of the history into the present illness section. Certainly, if you have a history of a heart catheterization or other heart procedure, mentioning the results earlier in the visit can help immensely. ◆

Chapter 4

Continuing Your Information Exchange

Now that we've covered the two most salient parts of the questioning, let's take a look at the rest of the doctor's sequence of questions.

STUDYING HISTORY

The history of your health should be divided into two sections: medical history and surgical history.

Medical History

Your medical history includes medical diagnoses such as hypertension, kidney disease, heart conditions, gastrointestinal disorders, neurological disease, and bone and joint problems, among many others. These represent chronic medical conditions or diagnoses that may be ongoing, treated and in remission, or cured.

It's best to communicate these conditions in reverse chronological order, listing active diagnoses first, then diagnoses in remission, and then prior conditions now considered remote or cured.

It's also helpful to comment on the type of treatment you received during each illness. For instance, for a diagnosis in remission such as Hodgkin's lymphoma, further relevant information may include mantle (chest wall) radiation, chemotherapy (with medication names), and length and dosage of chemotherapeutic treatments.

(Mantle radiation – radiation to the chest overlying the heart – can inflame the coronary arteries and, years later, result in obstructive coronary artery disease due to fibrosis and scarring.)

Therefore, a detailed list that includes treatment specifics presented in the form of an organized table or list can prove invaluable as an adjunct to the information gathered in the "chief complaint" and "history of present illness" sections. A truly complete medical history list permits the physician to scan the content without needing to ask further questions.

As a patient, your charge is to place your physician in a position to deliver the best possible health care. As you are no doubt starting to see, your biggest challenge is the limited time that's available for you to spend with your physician. This is why compiling a succinct history is superior to delivering an inch-thick stack of past medical records and expecting the physician to thoroughly review them, gather supplementary data, examine you, and record his findings – all within your visit's allotted 30 to 45 minutes.

However, if you don't have a medical background, you may not know how to accurately condense that inch-thick stack of records into a detailed list or table. If that's the case, what should you do?

For starters, recognize that simply having the information available at the time of your appointment is leaps and bounds ahead of the average patient. Even if you can't summarize the data, just by bringing the records with you, you've enhanced the quality of information exchange. Physicians are trained to sort through this information, although you should recognize that it may take extra valuable time.

Perhaps you have a relative or friend who has health-care experience and can sift through the mass of information. If not, you can still help the physician by making sure the papers are in order. I prefer the most recent papers first, as these data are more up-to-date and therefore more germane to the present visit.

Also, I find sticky notes helpful. Separate each hospital encounter or important testing result with a paper clip and use a sticky note to label each separate packet. For example, you might consider labeling a packet "1998 – Heart Bypass Surgery," another packet "1999 –

Pneumonia," and a third packet "2005 – Colonoscopy with Biopsy Results." Any type of systematic organization is helpful.

Consider my patient Paul, a 68-year-old retired machinist and avid coin collector. He came to see me because he was having recurring bouts of tightness in his chest and shortness of breath. He said both symptoms were much more pronounced when he mowed his lawn or played basketball in the driveway with his grandson.

After a detailed conversation with Paul, I realized that he might have coronary artery disease. Fortunately, he had brought a detailed medical history with him.

Items were listed separately in reverse chronological order and separated into three distinct categories: Active Diagnoses and Current Treatments, Diagnoses in Remission (ones that aren't active but have the potential to resurface), and Previous Conditions (ones in the past that aren't likely to recur).

ACTIVE DIAGNOSES AND CURRENT TREATMENTS

- **Hypertension.** Onset September 12, 1992
  - *Metoprolol 50 mg orally twice daily*
  - *Hydrochlorothiazide 25 mg orally once daily*
- **Rheumatoid arthritis.** Onset December 13, 1991
  - *Methotrexate 7.5 mg orally once per week*
- **Glaucoma.** Onset December 13, 1990
  - *Timolol Maleate two drops in each eye daily*
- **Insulin-requiring diabetes mellitus.** Onset August 10, 1989
  - *Humulin 70/30 10 units subcutaneously every morning*
- **Mitral valve prolapse.** Diagnosed by echocardiography January 10, 1989
  - *Antibiotics at the time of medical and dental procedures to prevent heart-valve infection*

DIAGNOSES IN REMISSION

- **Hodgkin's lymphoma.** Onset April 8, 1992
  - *Chest radiation, 15 sessions, treatment concluded July 10, 1992*

PREVIOUS CONDITIONS

- **Gastric ulcer.** Diagnosed by upper endoscopy at local physician office – April 17, 1998
  – *Prilosec 20 mg once daily for six months, no recurrence*
- **Pneumonia.** Hospitalized at Cleveland Clinic, Cleveland, Ohio, January 12-14, 1996
  – *Intravenous and oral antibiotics, 10 days total*
- **Diabetic ketoacidosis.** Hospitalized at Cleveland Clinic, Cleveland, Ohio, March 18-27, 1993
  – *Intensive care unit for three days, intravenous insulin and fluids*
- **Urinary tract infection with sepsis.** Hospitalized at Cleveland Clinic, Cleveland, Ohio, February 25-28, 1992
  – *Intravenous and oral antibiotics, seven days total*

The list painted a detailed picture of Paul's past health. When I examined it, I became even more concerned, seeing various clues to possible present and future issues.

As is true with most patients, each category was contributory. For example, in addition to the diabetes, I could immediately see other risk factors for coronary artery disease in his history – hypertension and chest radiation. In addition, I discovered that in August 1989, he had been diagnosed with insulin-requiring diabetes mellitus. Diabetes also significantly raises the odds of coronary artery obstruction. Knowing Paul's medical history was an important tool I used to evaluate his situation.

Surgical History

Surgical history is generally less complex than the medical history. Again, reverse chronological order is best.

List all potentially helpful details, such as the:

- Hospital's location
- Surgeon's name
- Operative findings
- Pathology results

DIABETES AND ITS RELATIONSHIP
TO HEART DISEASE

A person with diabetes has high blood-sugar (glucose) levels. This means that either the pancreas – which normally makes a hormone called insulin to help transport glucose into the body's cells – doesn't make enough insulin or the body can't use its own insulin as well as it should to help glucose get into the cells. This causes sugar to build up in the blood.

These elevated levels can cause serious health complications, including heart disease, impaired vision, kidney failure, and blockages in the legs and feet (called peripheral vascular disease).

Heart-related problems are caused when, over time, high glucose levels in the blood lead to changes in the blood-vessel wall. These changes predispose the diabetic to early atherosclerosis, which, in turn, makes the patient susceptible to ischemia (compromised blood flow and oxygen delivery to the heart) and heart attacks.

> Heart-related problems are caused when, over time, high glucose levels in the blood lead to changes in the blood-vessel wall.

Sometimes, the ischemia is not felt as chest pain because uncontrolled diabetes often causes neuropathy (nerve damage) that can blunt the typical pain response.

Diabetes is also associated with an increased tendency for platelets in the blood to clump together, as well as with elevations in certain blood lipids that also contribute to coronary artery blockage.

Although vision loss and kidney damage are two of the most feared diabetes-related health complications, cardiovascular disease is one of the most common and life-threatening ones. In fact, two of three people with diabetes die of either heart disease or stroke.

The good news is that a study known as the Diabetes Control and Complications Trial showed conclusively that intensive control of blood sugar lowers the long-term risk of cardiovascular-disease events.

Any complications such as an infection, adhesions, and blood clots should also be listed.

Paul's surgical history included:

Laparoscopic cholecystectomy (gallbladder removal). January 17, 1999
- Diagnosis: Chronic Cholecystitis
- Cleveland Clinic; Robert Smith, M.D.; Cleveland, Ohio

Thyroid biopsy. February 4, 1997
- Diagnosis: Benign Thyroid Tissue
- Cleveland Clinic; Robert Smith, M.D.; Cleveland, Ohio

Appendectomy. September 7, 1993
- Complicated by infection requiring two weeks of intravenous antibiotics
- Cleveland Clinic; Robert Smith, M.D.; Cleveland, Ohio

Right inguinal hernia repair. August 3, 1973
- Hospital unknown; William Jones, M.D.; Jackson, Mississippi

Staging laparotomy for Hodgkin's lymphoma. August 7, 1972
- Results not known
- Nashville General Hospital; James Carter, M.D.; Nashville, Tennessee

In this section, be as detailed as you can; it may provide your physician with valuable supplementary information pertaining to your chief complaint.

You don't have to use exact medical terminology. Perfect accuracy with medical terms and their spellings misses the point. It's fine to simply say, "My gallbladder was removed" or "They took out a piece of my intestine." The key is to communicate your information succinctly and accurately.

Because of Paul's chest discomfort and risk factors for coronary artery disease, he underwent a cardiac catheterization. A 90 percent blockage was found in the early portion of his left anterior descending coronary artery, the so-called "widow-maker."

He underwent successful intracoronary stent implantation and had complete resolution of his symptoms.

Medications

In your medical history file, you should include the name of every medication you take. This section should be divided into two parts: current medications and past medications. I find that the information is most easily and clearly presented in a tabular format. (See below.)

CURRENT MEDICATIONS

Your current medication list should include:

- The name of the medication
- The dose, usually in milligrams
- The dosing frequency (see "What Do Those Abbreviations Mean?" below)

WHAT DO THOSE ABBREVIATIONS MEAN?

Have you ever wondered what those abbreviations on your prescription stand for? They are all taken from Latin. It helps to know that "in die" means "a day," "cibum" means food, and "hora" means hour.

ABBREVIATION	LATIN PHRASE	WHAT IT MEANS
ac	ante cibum	Before meals
bid	bis in die	Twice a day
hs	hora somni	At bedtime
pc	post cibum	After meals
prn	pro re nata	As needed
q3h	quaque 3 hora	Every three hours
qd	quaque die	Every day
qid	quarter in die	Four times a day
tid	ter in die	Three times a day

- The date initiated
- Why the medication has been prescribed

Listing any perceived medication side effects can be helpful as they may be contributing to your current symptoms.

PAST MEDICATIONS

Your past medication list should include the same kind of information you use for your current medications. In addition, include the date you stopped using the medicine and the reason for termination.

In this section, it is particularly important to note any side effects so that you and your doctor can avoid that medication in the future.

Here's a good example of a complete medication list.

CURRENT MEDICATIONS

Name	Dose	Frequency	Date Started	Indication	Side Effects
Atenolol	25 mg	1 twice/day	1/06/98	Angina	Fatigue
Famotidine	20 mg	1 @ bedtime	12/09/97	Heartburn	None
Aspirin	325 mg	1 each a.m.	11/18/96	Coronary Disease	None
Simvastatin	20 mg	1 @ bedtime	11/09/95	High Lipids	None

PAST MEDICATIONS

Name	Dose/ Frequency	Date Started	Date Stopped	Indication	Side Effects
Propranolol	80 mg/ 1 twice/day	1/09/86	1/06/98	Angina	None
Gemfibrozil	600 mg/ 1 twice/day	4/08/88	4/28/97	High Lipids	None
Verapamil	80 mg/ 1 three times/day	2/19/88	5/18/95	Hypertension	Fatigue

PASS THE BOTTLE(S)

It's also important to bring your current medication bottles – with the actual pills – to your appointment. This way, your doctor can confirm your prepared list with the actual medications, ensuring accuracy.

Some patients aren't sure which drugs are which, or when to take them, and having the actual bottles and pills makes it easier to explain thoroughly.

INCLUDE VITAMINS AND OTHER SUPPLEMENTS OR HERBS

It's crucial that you let your doctor know whether you take vitamins, supplements, or herbal preparations. Although these generally don't require a prescription, they can be just as potent as a prescription medication.

Many have side effects and also may interact unsafely with your other medications. I can't stress how important it is to let your doctor know *everything* you are taking.

When I change a patient's medication dose or frequency, I often write the change on the existing bottle. That way, those pills still can be used when, say, the dose is doubled. With the cost of medicine today, this can be a real money-saver.

Also, I routinely place a mark on the bottle, especially if I'm stopping a medication. For senior patients who are taking a multitude of medications, putting a large "X" on the bottle is a clear way to alert them to stop taking it.

Another equally viable option is to simply discard the bottle at the time of the office visit. Many patients are reluctant to do so, in case they need to resume those medicines in the future. I advise against this, as each medication possesses a finite shelf life and there's a greater possibility of medication error.

I highly recommend keeping an up-to-date list of medications in your wallet at all times. Many medical facilities have cards available for this express purpose. If you can't easily find such cards, just use a 3-by-5 index card and fold it to fit in your wallet.

The list should include:

- The name of each medication
- Dosage amounts
- How often you take each medication

If you are away from home and require unanticipated medical care, a list of current medications could prove invaluable and perhaps even save your life.

If you are away from home and require unanticipated medical care, this list could prove invaluable and perhaps even save your life.

Allergies

Katherine, a 57-year-old nurse who had been recovering satisfactorily from a mild heart attack she suffered three years ago, recently mentioned a possible allergic reaction to one of her cardiac medications.

She had been taking the medication for several months. I was a bit suspicious, as an allergic reaction is mediated by the immune system and generally is observed shortly after the medication is first administered.

Allergic reactions may range from a slight itching or minor rash to a severe compromise in breathing, including swelling of the tongue and fatal anaphylaxis.

I asked Katherine, "Can you describe your allergic reaction for me?"

"The medicine seems to be giving me a headache, and I'm usually more tired after I take it," she said.

Katherine's comment was important, but in fact she was not allergic to the medication. Like many patients, she was mistakenly equating an allergic reaction and a nonallergic side effect. The latter isn't mediated by the immune system. Instead, it's an experienced effect of the medication. Common effects of cardiac medications include fatigue, headache, constipation, nausea, and flatulence.

Katherine was taking a long-acting form of nitroglycerin. This medication dilates blood vessels, including those in the brain. When I reduced her dosage slightly, her headaches were much more tolerable.

Allergies are an extremely important component of every health record. Knowing them can save your life.

MISSING MEDICATION INFORMATION
LEADS TO DELAYS, HASSLES

Knowing your current med-
ications is especially crucial
if you are having worrisome
symptoms. Your doctor may
want to consider adjusting
your medications to improve
how you feel.

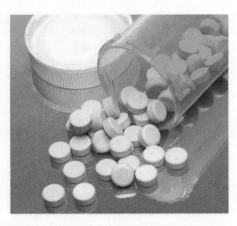

When my patients don't
know what medicines they're
taking – particularly patients
who may be taking several medications with a complicated dosing schedule
– I call their spouse or adult child from the exam room. If I can't reach a
family member by phone, I leave my e-mail address so they can e-mail me
a complete medication list.

Alternatively, the patient may go home and call in the information later
that day. I may then make some initial medication adjustments over the
phone, which is less than ideal (but still medically responsible because I've
seen the patient that day and I know his or her condition).

Since the patient is no longer in my office, I'll need to call the prescription into a pharmacy. The patient or a family member will then have to
leave home (or work) and pick up the medicine, which perhaps could have
been done more conveniently on the way home from the appointment,
with a written prescription in hand.

Obviously, this is a lot more inefficient than knowing your medications
up-front.

It also heightens the chance of errors: Someone may not hear accurately on the telephone; someone else may make a mistake reading
prescriptions off the bottle, or typing them into an e-mail. It's just easier
and safer to have all your medicine with you.

USING THE INTERNET: VISIT RELIABLE
SITES AND TALK TO YOUR DOCTOR

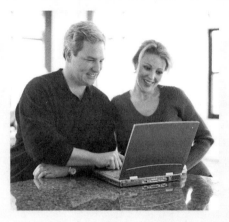

With the increased ease of obtaining medical information from the Internet, it is tempting to gather data about your symptoms, diagnoses, treatments, and medications. If you decide to do this, my best advice is to use only trustworthy and reliable Internet sources. Websites may raise a number of issues that may or may not apply to your condition and that can cause you a significant amount of anxiety and worry.

For example, a friend recently called me on a Saturday, very upset. She had received her echocardiogram report from her physician: It said only that she had a pericardial effusion and mitral valve leakage. Seeking an explanation on the Internet, she panicked after reading that pericardial effusion may be caused by a malignancy and that patients with mitral regurgitation (leakage) require valve surgery.

After reviewing the echocardiogram report the following Monday morning, I explained to her that she had a trivial pericardial effusion as well as a trivial leakage of her mitral valve, both insignificant findings. Because my friend did not have the medical background to realize that these findings were normal, she was unnecessarily distraught for two days.

The Internet can be helpful when used appropriately, but the patient who is immersed in his or her symptoms may not be the most objective person to sort out what is myth and what is reality.

For reliable, up-to-date information about cardiovascular topics, I highly recommend these websites: www.clevelandclinic.org (Cleveland Clinic) and www.americanheart.org (American Heart Association).

First-time medication reactions are difficult to predict and there-fore warrant advance patient education by the prescribing physician. Many medication allergies are detected in childhood. If you are a par-ent, note your children's allergies and communicate them to the school nurse. They should become a permanent component of your children's health files and should be shared with them as soon as they reach an age when they can understand the meaning and importance of an allergic reaction.

For your physician, prepare a list of your allergies with correspon-ding reactions. Here's how Katherine's appeared:

Medication	Allergic Reaction(s)
Penicillin	Hives
Sulfa	Shortness of breath, thick tongue
Iodinated x-ray dye	Red rash

Family Medical History

Certain illnesses are hereditary. Other conditions are identified with greater frequency or grouped within a family without necessarily being hereditary. For these reasons, your family medical history is an important part of your health record. Although it is typically gathered at the initial physician visit, a detailed preparation of this history in advance can eliminate the need for a time-consuming report during your appointment.

Knowing your family history can be highly beneficial. For instance, if I'm aware that a close relative of yours had coronary artery disease at an early age, I'll institute a more aggressive screening program than I might for someone without that family history. This means that if you *have* inherited that tendency, we have a much better chance of either preventing it or discovering and treating it early on.

Marshall's case is a good example of the importance of family his-tory. Marshall, a 68-year-old retired steel worker with three children and nine grandchildren, came to see me and my diagnosis was atrial fibrillation. Atrial fibrillation is a quivering, chaotic motion in the upper chambers of the heart (known as the atria). Atrial fibrillation, also called AF or Afib, is the most common sustained irregular heart rhythm in the United States.

The normal contraction of the two upper chambers of the heart followed by the two lower chambers causes an even, coordinated heartbeat that pumps blood from the heart out to the body between 60 to 100 beats per minute. In Afib, many electrical impulses begin chaotically and spread through the atria, causing a rapid heartbeat. Many individuals have Afib with no resulting problems, but chronic Afib can be associated with stroke, heart failure, and even death.

There's a long list of causes of atrial fibrillation, and it's sometimes difficult to pinpoint the exact cause. But it's the cardiologist's job to identify any factors that might be contributing to atrial fibrillation because these contributors are potentially treatable. Common contributors include:

- High blood pressure
- Excess caffeine intake
- Thyroid disorders
- Anemia
- Coexistent disease such as pneumonia or another infection that makes the heart electrically irritable
- Valvular heart disease
- Coronary artery disease

An echocardiogram is usually performed to rule out silent heart-valve leakage or other structural heart disease that might be causing the Afib. But during our appointment, Marshall mentioned that his father's doctor had once told him that his dad had had an abnormal thickening of the heart muscle. I knew that the condition – hypertrophic cardiomyopathy – had a tendency to cause cardiac arrhythmias and that its occurrence can be influenced by genetics and heredity. I was glad that Marshall had recalled the information and brought it to my attention. It's very important to identify this condition because a subset of the patients who have it are prone to sudden cardiac death as a result of severe arrhythmias.

Knowing the medical history of Marshall's father further honed my physical examination, and I was able to hear a murmur consistent with hypertrophic cardiomyopathy. I elicited the murmur by having Marshall perform a specific movement called the "Valsalva maneuver." The Valsalva maneuver can be done in one of two ways: The patient stands up from a squatting position or bears down as if he's going to have a bowel movement. These postures put a certain amount of stress on the heart and elicit a latent heart murmur that may not be audible during a regular examination.

The results of the Valsalva maneuver altered the sequence of my physical examination and made the cardiac examination more focused and detailed. I performed an echocardiogram shortly thereafter, which confirmed abnormal heart-muscle thickening, and referred Marshall to one of my electrophysiology colleagues to assess the potential for severe arrhythmias. Patients with severe arrhythmias benefit from implantation of a cardioverter-defibrillator to reduce their likelihood of sudden death.

Fortunately, Marshall had a mild form of hypertrophic cardiomyopathy. He was treated with medications and no further invasive procedures were required.

(A final note about hypertrophic cardiomyopathy: It has "incomplete penetrance," meaning that just because your first-degree relative has the condition, that doesn't mean that you will get it.)

WHO COUNTS AS "FAMILY"?

Most often, family history includes first-degree relatives, who are your

- Parents
- Siblings
- Children

Should a particular illness be pervasive – for instance, if your aunts, uncles, or grandparents have it – knowing that can also be helpful.

A good format that I like to follow for a family medical history can be found on the next page. When you present the family's history like this, the physician can scan it quickly and with ease. She'll look for

Family Member	Age	Illness	Age of Onset	Age at Death
Father	65	Hypertension	64	N/A
		Migraine headaches	63	
		Hyperlipidemia	62	
Mother	62	Osteoarthritis	58	N/A
		Diabetes mellitus	56	
		Glaucoma	55	
Maternal G'mother		Myocardial infarction	82	82
		Diabetes mellitus	76	
		Glaucoma	66	
		Osteoarthritis	62	
Paternal G'mother	N/A	Myocardial infarction	64	64
Brother	42	None	N/A	N/A
Brother	41	Hypertension	38	N/A
Daughter	18	Mitral valve prolapse	16	N/A
Son	16	None	N/A	N/A

diseases that span generations, such as hypertension, diabetes mellitus, premature coronary artery disease, and malignancies.

If you know your relative's age when the illness began, it's important to include this information. For example, a patient whose first-degree relative was diagnosed with CAD before the age of 55 is considered at risk for the development of premature coronary artery disease. On the other hand, if coronary disease is identified in an octogenarian, it's a much less powerful risk factor for the younger generation.

Also note that under the "illness" category, illnesses are listed in reverse chronological order. As in the medical history section, this provides systematic order to the presentation.

Social History

Your social history comprises several important components, including:

- Social habits
- Occupations (present and past)
- Education level
- Marital status
- Number of children

Gynecological history (if relevant), childhood illnesses (if not previously mentioned), immunization status, and exercise habits may also be included. Less common but appropriate information may include your travel history – particularly if you travel to underdeveloped countries – as well as exposure to toxins and illnesses.

Let's address each of these categories in more detail.

SOCIAL HABITS

Social habits include tobacco use, alcohol use, and illicit drug use. For each, record the beginning and ending dates (if applicable) and the average quantity or amount used. For example, tobacco use may be specified by age of onset, age of quitting, and average use in packs per day. A similar attempt at quantifying alcohol use and other substances is appropriate.

Here's a look at a sample table that depicts social habits:

Habit	Age of Onset	Age of Cessation	Average Daily Consumption
Cigarettes	22	42	2 packs
Alcohol	none	n/a	n/a
Drugs (marijuana)	19	25	1 or 2 "cigarettes" per month

OCCUPATIONS

Current and past occupations may provide a number of health clues. For instance, if you've had a desk job for the past 30 years, your lifestyle will be sedentary compared to that of an aerobics instructor or firefighter.

Working in a nuclear power plant or in a fertilizer factory may reveal past and ongoing toxic exposures. Past occupations also are relevant and may provide insight regarding radiation exposure that occurred at a time when regulations were less stringent.

Again, recording the occupation in a tabular format and in reverse chronological order is ideal.

Occupation	Starting Age	Ending Age	Exposures
Accountant	22	present	none
Lifeguard	16	21	excessive sun
Camp Counselor	14	16	none

EDUCATION LEVEL

This isn't an essential component of the health record but should be included for completeness. If the physician identifies a particular area of patient expertise, this may permit a discussion of greater depth. It also may help identify an area of common interest between the physician and patient, and serve as a means of introduction and rapport-building, particularly during the first meeting.

The listing can be brief:

- *Graduated from Rocky River High School, Rocky River, Ohio, 1968*

MARITAL STATUS AND NUMBER OF CHILDREN

Similarly, these are nonessential components of the health record but should be obtained for completeness. Understanding who composes the immediate family is important should the health-care discussion involve additional family members. And because certain health problems are hereditary, it may be important for other family members to be screened for similar afflictions.

Again, the listing can be brief:

- Currently married to first wife of 28 years
- Son, 24, alive and well
- Daughter, 18, alive and well

GYNECOLOGICAL HISTORY

This section addresses childbirth history, frequency and timing of menstrual cycles, birth control methods, and the dates and results of your most recent mammogram and Pap smear. If you've had gynecologic surgical procedures, it's more helpful to place them in the earlier "past surgeries" section.

This table may appear as follows:

Year of Pregnancy	Pregnancy Outcome	Mode of Delivery	Complications
1961	live birth	vaginal	none
1959	live birth	vaginal	Hypertension

Menstrual History	Age of Onset	Age of Cessation	Frequency	Birth Control
	12	ongoing 28 days	regular	none

Mammogram Date	Result	Pap Smear Date	Result
April 28, 2000	normal	April 16, 2006	normal

Other information you might consider including:

Childhood Illness	Age	Hospitalization Required/Length	Complications
Rheumatic Fever	6	Yes, 7 days	Heart Murmur
Strep Throat	4, 6, 9	no	none known

Immunization Type	Date of Last Administration
Tetanus Toxoid	June 28, 1996
Influenza Vaccine	October 23, 2000

Exercise Type	Frequency	Duration
Treadmill	4 times per week	30 minutes
Free Weights	3 times per week	30 minutes

Travel Destination	Year	Duration	Immunizations/ Medications Before Travel
England	2000	2 weeks	none
Japan	1998	1 week	none
India	1998	10 days	yes (Hepatitis A vaccine)

ELECTRONIC MEDICAL RECORDS

The advent of the electronic medical record – a computer-based copy of a person's entire health-care history – has greatly benefited both patients and physicians. Once the aforementioned historical data are entered, they are in your chart permanently.

Many physicians' offices and hospitals belong to the same health system and use the same electronic medical records. So information about previous appointments, medical and surgical histories, and an up-to-date medication list are readily available. All that is required is periodic updating at the time of your subsequent appointments.

An electronic chart allows the physician to communicate with you in a more timely manner. It reduces telephone traffic and allows you to participate in your own health care by being able to have results sent to you electronically with explanations from the treating doctor.

In addition to the enhanced precision and ease of communication of patient information, the electronic medical record also has printing capabilities. Therefore, at the end of each of your appointments, an appointment summary can be printed for you to take home, including a list of your current medications.

With electronic charts, there is a "break-in" period for both the patient and the physician. Entering these data initially can be quite time-consuming and may extend your visit.

Having an electronic medical record does *not* mean that you need not bother to prepare for your physician visit. Instead, after the first visit, it permits the physician to focus less on your history and medications and more on your current concern. It allows you to focus less on historical details at the time of your subsequent appointments and, instead, to direct your efforts toward your chief complaint and present illness sections. Both these scenarios still require the careful advanced preparation discussed in previous chapters.

Review of Systems

The review of systems is a catch-all category. As its name suggests, it serves as a general review of all health systems.

An easy, logical approach to this section of your written summary is to move downward from your head to your toes. The following list includes the major review of systems components and notes possible relevant symptoms and diagnoses.

General overview: Weight gain or loss, perception of your general state of health, sweats, fevers, chills

Head: Headaches, dizziness, lightheadedness, injury

Eyes: Pain, tearing, glasses, diminished vision, blind spots, cataracts, glaucoma, trauma

Ears: Diminished hearing, hearing aids, infection, discharge, wax build-up

Nose: Excessive discharge or drainage, reduced smell, pain, difficulty breathing, bleeding

Mouth: Excessive or reduced salivation, halitosis, dentures, growths or tumors, pain, altered sense of taste, bleeding gums or swelling

Neck: Stiffness, pain, swollen glands or lymph nodes, thyroid enlargement

Lungs: Shortness of breath, wheezing, fluid collection, pneumonia, bronchitis, pain with breathing, cough, coughing blood, tuberculosis or exposure to tuberculosis, fever, night sweats

Heart: Chest discomfort, palpitations, fluid retention, near-fainting or fainting, shortness of breath, less tolerance for exercise, hypertension, heart murmurs, phlebitis, leg-muscle cramps/burning with walking

Gastrointestinal system: Appetite change, difficulty swallowing, painful swallowing, heartburn, nausea, vomiting, constipation, diarrhea, change in stool (caliber, consistency, or color), blood in stool, abdominal pain, jaundice, hemorrhoids, flatulence

Genitourinary system: Increased frequency or urgency of urination, increased urination at night, blood in the urine, reduced volume of urine, stones/sediment in the urine, infections, urinary dribbling, incontinence, genital sores, discharge, venereal disease, libido change, impotence, vaginal discharge, excessive menstrual flow, painful intercourse, postmenopausal bleeding

Skin/Breast: Rash, itching, pigmentation, moisture or dryness, texture, changes in hair growth or loss, nail changes, breast lumps, breast tenderness, breast swelling, nipple discharge

Musculoskeletal system: Pain, swelling, reduced range of joint motion, muscle weakness, muscle shrinkage, muscle cramps

Neurologic/Psychiatric systems: Tremor, coordination, paralysis, weakness, gait disturbance, seizures, stroke, speech difficulties, memory difficulties, altered sensation, numbness, anxiety disorder, panic disorder, depression, hallucinations, altered perceptions

Allergies/Immune system: Rashes; reactions to medications (prescription and nonprescription), foods, previous blood transfusions, insects; immunodeficiency

Blood: Anemia, easy bruising, tendencies toward blood-clotting, abnormal blood-clotting

Lymphatic system: Enlarged lymph nodes, tender lymph nodes

Endocrine system: Intolerance to heat or cold, excessive water requirements, excessive/frequent urination, thyroid enlargement, abnormal height (tall or short), excessive secondary hair growth

Once you and your doctor have discussed your past and present health, it's time to pursue your diagnosis and treatment. ◆

Chapter 5

What You Should Know about Diagnostic Testing

Now that you're prepared for your first meeting with your cardiologist, it's time to become familiar with the testing procedures that he may recommend. It's likely that you've heard about many of these, but perhaps you don't know quite what to expect. Invariably, your doctor will perform one or more of these tests.

Knowing about these tests ahead of time should improve your relationship with your cardiologist since you'll be better able to understand the need for the test, know what to expect, and be able to ask pertinent questions when you get the results.

THE BASICS

There are several main tests that cardiologists order frequently: the electrocardiogram (EKG/ECG), stress-testing, and echocardiogram (echo). We'll look at these three first and then expand into the tests that may follow, especially when results of the initial tests are abnormal.

Electrocardiogram

An electrocardiogram detects and records the heart's electrical activity – when and where its electrical signals are generated. It shows the rate of your heartbeat (fast or slow) and its rhythm (steady or irregular).

The test is easy to perform, painless, and risk-free. Ten electrodes (wires) are attached to your body using disposable sticky pads. One is placed on each arm and leg, and six are placed across the center and left side of your chest. The electrocardiograph records your heart's activity for a minute or so. Then your cardiologist can readily interpret the results.

When considered in conjunction with the patient's history and physical exam, the electrocardiogram serves as an excellent screening tool for cardiovascular disease. It permits a rapid assessment of the heart rhythm and heart-chamber sizes, and may record evidence of heart damage from a previous heart attack. Your doctor may identify certain prolonged electrical intervals that may reflect abnormal serum chemistries, such as potassium and calcium levels, that affect the heart.

Despite these capabilities, the electrocardiogram isn't foolproof. Normal results don't exclude structural heart disease with 100 percent certainty. Remember, the EKG assesses your heart at rest. Occasionally, an abnormal recording may instead represent a "normal variant," whereby a finding may suggest structural heart disease that further testing will rule out. Despite these occasional shortcomings, the electrocardiogram remains an outstanding test because of its availability, absence of risk, low cost, and immediacy of results.

Remember Robert, whose story we've been following? Because of the racing heartbeat he reported, his doctor first had him undergo an EKG. When the arrhythmia didn't occur during the test, Robert went on to Holter monitoring (described below).

Stress Test

A stress test represents a noninvasive (external) way to assess whether there is a blocked or narrowed coronary artery that limits blood flow. You are likely to have this type of test if your cardiologist suspects the presence of flow-limiting coronary artery obstructions.

We've seen that the cardiac muscle's blood-pumping function depends on oxygen-rich blood supplied by the coronary arteries. Atherosclerosis (the plaque that blocks arteries) remains a major health concern worldwide and is the cause of many heart attacks (myocardial infarctions) and, sometimes, sudden cardiac death.

Typically, before a stress test will reveal an abnormality, at least 60 percent to 70 percent of the inner channel of a coronary artery must be blocked. This is called "flow-limiting blockage" or "flow-limiting stenosis." Lesser blockages may not show up on this type of test.

SUPPLY AND DEMAND

The cardiac stress test employs the simple concept of supply and demand. Even if there is coronary artery blockage, under most circumstances when the body is less active, its oxygen demand is lower and the heart will continue to receive an adequate amount of blood. Therefore, the heart's oxygen supply is meeting demand.

But when the oxygen requirement is heightened, as it is during exercise, the reduced supply of blood doesn't meet the demand. This supply/demand mismatch leaves the heart with an inadequate supply of oxygen, which is called "myocardial ischemia."

HOW IT'S DONE

During a stress test, you'll walk or jog on a treadmill as its speed and incline are gradually increased according to your exercise capabilities. Medical professionals monitor your blood pressure and electrocardiogram data every few minutes. The test puts enough stress on the heart to assess cardiac blood flow and oxygen delivery to the heart muscle.

A stress test will show:

1. How well you meet the expected exercise capacity for your age.
2. Whether your symptoms, such as chest discomfort or undue shortness of breath, are provoked under stress (suggesting artery blockage).
3. Whether there is a gradual increase in heart rate while a normal rhythm is maintained, as there should be, and whether this is followed by a rapid decline in heart rate after exercising (normal heart-rate recovery).
4. Assessment of blood pressure at rest and during activity. Blood pressure should increase gradually throughout the test.
5. Analysis of electrocardiographic data, taken when you begin exercise (the baseline) and at peak exercise. A segment on the electrocardiogram called the "ST segment" should not go below the baseline. If it does, it may reflect impaired heart-blood flow (myocardial ischemia).

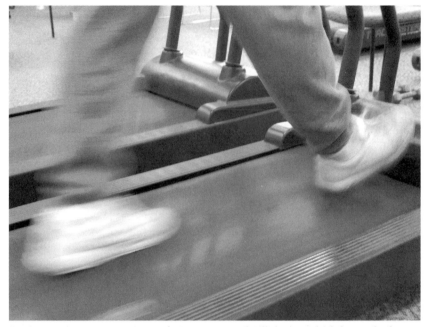

During a stress test, a patient exercises on a treadmill during which heart rhythm, heart rate, and blood pressure are continuously monitored. In addition, the patient receives surveillance monitoring during a program of cardiac rehabilitation.

Exercise stress tests can be combined with either echocardiography or nuclear imaging ("scintigraphy") tests to enhance their diagnostic accuracy.

If you have a highly abnormal stress test, it's likely that you'll need to undergo a heart catheterization to define more precisely the number, location, and extent of your coronary artery obstructions.

Ambulatory Blood-Pressure Monitoring

Sometimes a patient's blood pressure is elevated in the physician's office because of the anxiety surrounding the appointment, a condition termed "white-coat hypertension." As a result, the doctor may not be able to tell whether the patient's blood pressure would be normal under daily conditions outside of the medical office.

In this situation and in other circumstances when it is important to obtain a highly accurate blood-pressure reading, ambulatory blood-pressure monitoring may be performed.

An ambulatory blood-pressure monitor is attached to the upper arm by means of a standard blood-pressure cuff. At approximately every 15 to 30 minutes, the blood-pressure cuff automatically inflates and the value is recorded.

A small waist pack the size of a transistor radio is attached to the blood-pressure cuff by small hoses or tubes. This waist pack, which is battery-powered, records the blood pressure for a period of up to 24 hours. This feature provides the physician frequent blood-pressure checks throughout the day. It also permits the recording of these blood pressures during varying levels of activity, including exercise and sleep.

Obtaining recordings during sleep can be quite helpful as blood pressure normally decreases or "dips" during deep sleep. The lack of this "nocturnal dip" can lend greater certainty to the diagnosis of hypertension.

Ambulatory blood-pressure monitoring has no known risks except for periodic discomfort during inflation of the blood-pressure cuff and recording. Also, the intermittent inflation of the blood-pressure cuff may cause the patient some difficulty in sleeping.

CARDIAC IMAGING TESTS

Echocardiogram

An echocardiogram is a sound-wave (ultrasound) test that images the heart. It typically takes 30 minutes or less. You lie mainly on your left side, while several electrodes attached to your chest record your heart rhythm. A small amount of transducer gel is applied to the echocardiogram probe (it resembles a microphone in shape and size) to facilitate transmission of echocardiographic images, ensuring optimal clarity for the doctor's interpretation.

Similar to the electrocardiogram, an echocardiogram is readily obtainable, results are immediately available, and there's no known risk to you. In addition, you won't experience any discomfort.

An echocardiogram permits precise assessment of the sizes of your cardiac chambers. It also assesses your "pericardial space." The peri-

cardium is the sac containing a nominal amount of fluid that lubri-
cates the heart's surface. When abnormality is present, your doctor
can readily visualize fluid accumulation beyond normal levels.

An echocardiogram also permits assessment of how your heart
pumps, allowing the interpreter to classify it as either normal or
weakened to mild, moderate, or severe degrees. Also, heart-muscle
weakening can be classified as regional (abnormal in a discrete location) or global (evenly distributed throughout the heart muscle).
Regional heart-muscle dysfunction typically represents a previous
heart attack overlying a particular coronary artery distribution, whereas global heart-muscle dysfunction can be seen, for instance, in
patients with longstanding, poorly controlled high blood pressure.

Another outstanding virtue of an echocardiogram is its ability to
assess all four cardiac valves more effectively than any other available
technology. One technique (Doppler color-flow imaging) is especially
useful for identifying valvular heart disease, such as regurgitation.

An echocardiogram also allows your doctor to estimate the pressure
within each heart chamber. In abnormal situations such as valvular
heart disease and/or heart-muscle weakening, heart pressures may
be elevated, suggesting the need to begin and/or adjust medication
dosages.

Starting medication use or adjusting present dosages can lower
these pressures, resulting in an enhanced sense of well-being,
improved activity level, and less stress and strain on the heart.

Stress Echocardiogram

To enhance the diagnostic reliability of stress-testing, cardiac imaging
is often performed simultaneously with treadmill exercise. During a
stress (exercise) echocardiogram, an echocardiogram is performed
first while you are at rest, as described above. Then you are asked to
exercise on a treadmill to your maximum ability. (See "Stress Test,"
page 60.)

Immediately after exercise, without a cool-down period, you're
taken to the echocardiogram exam table (right next to the treadmill)
for a post-exercise echocardiogram. The post-exercise echocardio-

gram assesses your regional and global heart-pumping function ("contractility") during your peak exercise heart rate.

Under normal circumstances, the heart's function after exercise should demonstrate symmetrical and vigorous enhancement of its pumping function. A reduction in this pumping function that is localized to one territory of the heart reliably predicts significant coronary artery blockage and impaired delivery of oxygen to the heart muscle.

When several areas show reduced heart-pumping capacity after exercise, it is highly indicative of more than one coronary artery blockage, often termed "multivessel coronary artery disease."

Dobutamine Echocardiogram

Some patients aren't able to exercise on a treadmill. If you're in this group, your doctor can perform dobutamine echocardiography, in which you are administered a medication that will stress your heart in a way that is similar to exercising.

To raise your heart rate in a gradual, controlled way, dobutamine, a medication similar in effect to adrenaline, is slowly administered through an intravenous line. As your heart rate increases, echocardiogram images are obtained and recorded, and compared side by side.

Under normal circumstances, the heart pumps more strongly and responds in a symmetrical fashion as its rate increases in response to the dobutamine infusion. In disease states such as coronary artery disease, however, one portion of the heart may not contract as strongly as other portions in response to the dobutamine. This usually signals a coronary blockage and oxygen deprivation of the heart muscle in that region.

Similar to exercise echocardiography, a reduction in heart function in several areas following dobutamine infusion typically signals multivessel coronary blockage.

Nuclear Imaging

Nuclear stress-testing can be an extremely useful technique for assessing blood flow in the coronary arteries. It involves the injection of a radioactive "tracer" into the body, followed by a reading of its gamma-ray emissions taken with a gamma camera. The tracer is given in a tiny amount that doesn't harm the body. It travels to the heart and, by way of the coronary arteries, concentrates in the heart muscle.

The tracer "lights up" in the parts of the heart where blood is flowing (cardiac perfusion). These parts are often called "hot spots." Areas of the heart that are dark and emit no tracer activity show where the supply of blood is inadequate. Dark areas are often called "cold spots."

Nuclear imaging (also called radionuclide imaging and nuclear scintigraphy) may be performed on a treadmill or – as with the pharmacologic echocardiography stress test described earlier – by using a medication to stress the heart in those who cannot exercise. For nuclear stress tests, the intravenous medication adenosine is often chosen. This medication normally dilates the heart's arteries, enhancing blood flow to unobstructed areas of heart muscle. Adenosine cannot cause dilation of the coronary arteries in the presence of advanced blockage and so does not affect blood flow to oxygen-deprived heart muscle. This creates mismatched blood flow and thus generates the "hot" and "cold" spots.

An exercise nuclear stress test couples a routine exercise stress test performed on a treadmill with a small amount of radioactive tracer injected intravenously during the peak of exercise.

An exercise nuclear stress test couples a routine exercise stress test performed on a treadmill with a small amount of radioactive tracer injected intravenously during the peak of exercise. After exercising, you lie still on a table for several minutes while an external camera records heart blood flow indicated by emissions of gamma rays from the injected material. These pictures are compared to a similar set of pictures taken while you were at rest.

If the perfusion of the heart muscle is normal at rest but abnormal during exercise, this is a strong indication of myocardial ischemia. If the images show abnormal perfusion at rest and during exercise, this most often indicates heart-muscle damage and scarring caused by a heart attack.

Cardiac Catheterization (Coronary Angiogram)

If your doctor suspects that you have coronary artery disease, he may recommend further diagnostic testing in the form of a cardiac catheterization. This procedure is performed under sterile conditions in a special radiology suite with real-time x-ray guidance, known as "fluoroscopy." (The suite is often called the "cardiac catheterization laboratory," or "cath lab" for short.)

The test involves advancing a tiny catheter to your coronary arteries and injecting them with dye that will show whether the arteries are blocked. Sometimes, if a blockage is discovered, the same procedure will continue with treatment to unblock the artery.

Here is a more detailed explanation.

Your groin area is covered, shaved, and scrubbed with a sterile solution. Next, a small amount of numbing medication is inserted below your skin in the region of your upper leg fold, over your femoral artery. The doctor (a specialist termed an "invasive cardiologist") inserts a small needle into the femoral artery through the numbed area.

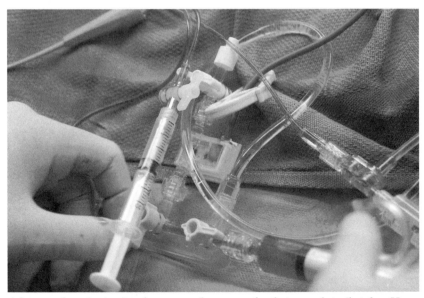

A heart catheterization involves a complex array of catheters and sterile tubes. Here, the patient's blood is combined with intra-arterial contrast dye before being injected into the coronary arteries. By rendering the arteries opaque, the dye reveals where the arteries are blocked.

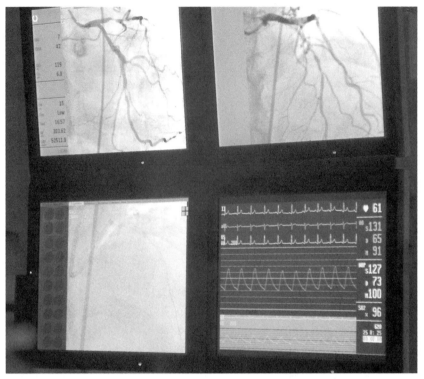

During a heart catheterization, the coronary arteries are depicted on monitors. The upper left quadrant demonstrates several narrowings or blockages. The lower right quadrant demonstrates the heart-rate, blood-pressure, and heart-rhythm recordings on a continuous basis.

A wire is inserted through this small needle to gain access to your femoral artery. Once the wire is in place, a small plastic catheter, known as an "introducer," is carefully advanced over the wire, and the wire is removed. (A catheter is a long, preshaped hollow tube approximately the diameter of a piece of cooked spaghetti.) The introducer is temporarily sewn into place.

The introducer has a one-way valve, permitting the introduction of additional catheters into your bloodstream while preventing backflow bleeding. Because there are no pain-sensitive nerves within the blood vessels, there is no discomfort when a catheter is introduced.

Under careful x-ray fluoroscopic guidance, the catheter is slowly advanced through the introducer into your femoral artery and up your aorta into your chest in the vicinity of your heart. Its journey takes it to the openings of your left and right coronary artery, known as your coronary ostia.

Once positioned at the entry point of a coronary artery, a small amount of radio-opaque x-ray dye is injected into the catheter. The dye travels the length of the catheter from your groin to the heart, and exits at its end. The dye mixes with the blood entering the coronary artery.

By observing (on a monitor) the behavior of this dye-and-blood mixture as it travels through the artery, the physician can assess the presence and severity of coronary artery blockages. He does this by noting whether the mixture travels smoothly through the artery or whether it is detained or completely stopped by rough spots or lumps representing blockages. In normal circumstances, the inside channels of coronary arteries are smooth tubes devoid of any such rough spots.

In some situations, the blockages may be hazy and therefore their severity may be difficult to quantify. Because the procedure is being recorded in real time under fluoroscopy, the pictures obtained on the angiogram are digitally recorded and can be replayed for subsequent careful analysis.

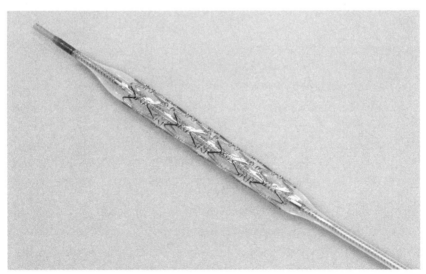

An intracoronary stent, located on a central catheter. Note the scaffold-type latticework. Once deployed, the stent will displace and buttress any atherosclerotic plaque to the vessel wall. This reduces the likelihood of future impairment of blood flow in the coronary artery.

Coronary artery disease doesn't follow a specific pattern. While blockages are frequently seen at the branch points of coronary artery blood vessels, they can occur at any point within the coronary artery system. In fact, under severe circumstances, coronary arteries can appear "diffusely" narrowed throughout their entirety, making it difficult to discern the location of the the most severe blockage.

Alternatively, situations can arise in which the coronary arteries resemble a string of pearls, displaying a succession of severe individual blockages.

Both these patterns may be amenable to treatment with coronary stents or coronary artery bypass surgery. Each case is individual and depends upon the number and pattern of the blockages coupled with the size of the coronary arteries. Your case is best discussed with your cardiologist.

Medications to relieve symptoms, reduce heart workload, and improve blood flow are uniformly administered.

Cardiac Computed Tomography (Cardiac CT)

You've probably heard of a CT or CAT scan. A traditional CT scan combines many x-ray images to produce cross-sectional views of the body.

Cardiac CT uses CT technology with intravenous (IV) contrast material (dye) to image the entire cardiac anatomy, coronary circulation, and great vessels (the aorta and pulmonary arteries).

During the test, you lie supine on a scanning table. Electrodes are placed on your chest and an IV line is placed in your arm. You will be asked to raise your arms over your head. The scanning table then glides you into a donut-shaped scanner. The contrast agent may cause a warm sensation as it is put into the IV. Images are collected within 15 seconds, and the test is over.

Computer processing and image manipulation render a 3-D image that clearly defines the spatial relationships between contiguous cardiac structures. If you're facing invasive procedures, this information can prove invaluable.

For example, if you have developed progressive blockages since your first bypass and if you're scheduled for a second bypass procedure, the cardiac CT permits precise localization of your original bypass grafts.

When your surgeon reenters your chest cavity, he will be aware of the location of the preexisting bypass grafts, significantly reducing the possibility of injury to them.

Perhaps the most common reason for doctors to perform a cardiac CT is to assess the aorta. In patients with aortic aneurysm and aortic dissection, the test allows for direct visualization of the aorta in its entirety, including precise measurements at every level. (See Chapter 6 for details on aortic aneurysm and dissection.)

This can be extremely helpful in an urgent case when a dissection or aneurysm is suspected.

Cardiac CT is also used to follow known aortic abnormalities to monitor for changes, such as enlargement.

Computed Tomography Angiogram (CT Angio, CTA)

Another type of cardiac CT is the computed tomography angiogram, also known as "CT angio" and "CTA." It is a great way to evaluate the coronary arteries while avoiding the invasiveness of a cardiac catheterization.

For this procedure, a small intravenous line is started in your arm. Medications, most often in the form of IV beta blockers and a nitroglycerin tablet placed under your tongue, are administered to slow your heart rate and dilate your coronary arteries to enhance the quality of the images. X-ray dye is also injected through the IV line.

X-rays pass through the body and are picked up by special detectors. Detailed images are acquired within seconds, and results are available for interpretation shortly thereafter, once they've received the same kind of computer processing and image manipulation as is done in cardiac CT.

When the results are normal, CTA reliably excludes the presence of significant coronary atherosclerosis.

CTA can detect mild degrees of coronary atherosclerosis. This information is quite useful because your doctor can recommend lifestyle changes or medical treatment that can prevent these atherosclerotic plaques from developing into a serious problem at a later date.

DRAWBACKS OF CTA

CTA may reveal calcified plaque. The calcified plaque often casts a shadow, which can complicate the physician's assessment of blockage severity.

If the patient has had a stent placed in the artery, that also casts a shadow and at times precludes the assessment of restenosis (renarrowing) within the stent.

Despite these limitations, the way cardiac CTA visualizes the coronary arteries, including inside stents, is improving. Someday it may replace the need for a heart catheterization – a benefit, since CTA is less invasive and therefore less risky than catheterization.

WHICH IS BETTER: CTA OR CARDIAC CATH?

Coronary CTA can be performed much more quickly than a cardiac catheterization and it has less potential for risk and discomfort, as well as a negligible recovery time. However, cardiac catheterization remains the "gold standard" for detecting coronary artery stenosis.

At present, coronary CTA is best employed as a screening procedure assessing coronary artery blockages. When symptoms are present that strongly suggest blockage, or if the patient is having an acute heart attack, a cardiac catheterization is still the way to go.

This is a fast-moving area that has made remarkable technological advances. Expect these recommendations to evolve over time – perhaps in the near future.

Cardiac Magnetic Resonance Imaging (MRI)

Cardiac MRI is a noninvasive imaging procedure that is commonly performed to examine the heart's structure and function. Unlike CT, it doesn't require x-ray radiation but instead relies upon magnetic resonance to provide images of the heart's chambers, valves, and vessels. (Patients with metal implants such as pacemakers, defibrillators, brain aneurysm clips, and orthopedic joint replacements can't undergo MRI because of its powerful magnetic field.)

An IV is started and a special imaging agent (gadolinium) is administered. You lie on a special table that slides into a donut-shaped scanner. Being in the enclosed MRI cylinder may produce a feeling of confinement, although some newer machines minimize this feeling. If you are extremely anxious at the thought of being in an enclosed space, you may be able to take a sedative. Ask beforehand.

As with cardiac CT, MRI provides excellent imaging of the cardiac chambers and surrounding chest structures. It can assess heart and valve function with greater precision than cardiac CT, whereas both tests provide aortic imaging of similar quality.

If you have impaired kidney function, cardiac MRI would be preferable to cardiac CT. This is because gadolinium doesn't lead to possible (albeit infrequent) kidney effects as does the iodinated x-ray dye used for CT scans.

HEART-RHYTHM TESTS

Holter Monitoring

Holter monitoring (named for its inventor, Dr. Norman Holter) is a means to record the heart rhythm over a length of time, usually 24 to 48 hours, while the patient goes about a normal day at work and at home. It is quite useful when someone, such as our friend Robert, is suspected to have a heart-rhythm abnormality that doesn't occur during a doctor's visit or goes undetected on an ECG.

To undergo the monitoring, several electrodes were attached to Robert's chest and connected to a small waist pack the size of a transistor radio. For 48 hours, the monitor recorded every heartbeat.

Robert was given a diary in which to record the type and character of each symptom as well as his activity level and the time of day. In this way, Robert's perceived abnormal symptoms could be pinpointed on the heart-rhythm recording. The irregular rhythm happened just once during the two days he wore the monitor.

Once Robert had turned in his Holter monitor, a trained technician assessed the minimum, maximum, and average heart rates, and evaluated the possible presence of abnormal heart rhythms. Dr. Smith received a report of the findings.

As Dr. Smith suspected, Robert's heart rate was caused by an atrial rhythm disorder. In Robert's case, this was atrial flutter, a fast heart rate that starts in the heart's upper chambers and is transmitted to the lower chambers. Because atrial flutter can occur in people with preexisting heart conditions such as pericarditis, coronary artery disease, heart-muscle weakening, heart-muscle thickening, and valvular heart disease, Dr. Smith ordered an echocardiogram and stress test for Robert. After reviewing the results, Dr. Smith assured Robert that there was no evidence of these other abnormalities.

The Holter monitor can also detect silent heart-rhythm disturbances that may be abnormal and life-threatening, such as ventricular tachycardia. Such information is invaluable since it can help dictate further testing and treatment.

At the other end of the spectrum, some patients who are experiencing what they believe to be heart-rhythm abnormalities may undergo Holter monitoring and discover that no arrhythmias are to be found.

Event Recorders and Loop Recorders

Because Holter monitors are typically worn only for 24 to 48 hours, they may not detect heart-rhythm disturbances in patients with infrequent arrhythmias. In such instances, event recorders, which can be worn for up to 30 days at a time, may be helpful.

Instead of a continuous recording, an event recorder is patient-activated, recording heart rhythms only when the patient experiences his or her symptoms and pushes a button.

The event recorder has a transtelephonic component that allows the patient to transmit the suspected heart-rhythm abnormality over the telephone (using a land line, not a cell phone) with real-time interpretation.

If something serious is discovered, this information is instantaneously transmitted to the physician, who can contact the patient and act upon the results accordingly.

An implantable event recorder, also known as a loop recorder, is a newer technology. The loop recorder is much smaller than a pacemaker and is implanted under the skin below the collar bone. This device records the heart rhythm for up to several months for those patients in whom a Holter monitor or an event recorder has not been able to detect abnormal heart rhythms.

Ordinarily, loop recorders aren't used because few patients require one, but they can be extremely helpful for those patients who are convinced that they have an abnormal heart rhythm despite negative results on the Holter monitor and event recorder, or in those patients who have extremely infrequent symptoms.

Electrophysiology (EP) Study

An electrophysiology (EP) study is an invasive procedure similar to a cardiac catheterization, but it is designed to check your heart's electrical system rather than the coronary arteries.

The groin area is shaved and prepared in a sterile manner similar to preparation for a heart catheterization. A catheter with an electrode on the tip is introduced into the bloodstream and guided to the heart. The electrode is connected to an ECG machine.

Once inside the heart, the catheter precisely measures the heart's electrical activity and pathways. In addition, the electrophysiologist conducting the test will stimulate the heart in certain ways. This will help him or her see how well the heart's electrical system is functioning.

Treatment with an ablation catheter that destroys the abnormal electrical circuit sometimes happens immediately after a problem area is detected.

An EP study can often be extremely valuable in uncovering abnormal and potentially life-threatening heart-rhythm abnormalities that are not recorded by electrocardiography, Holter monitoring, or event recording.

By uncovering these rhythm disturbances, curative ablation can be offered. In situations where ablation is not possible, such as numerous rhythm disturbances emanating from a variety of heart locations, the best choice is to have a cardiac defibrillator implanted. ◈

Chapter 6

Cardiovascular Diagnoses and Their Treatments

This chapter gives you an overview of some of the major cardiovascular diagnoses, how they are detected, and what may comprise their treatments. I believe that the more you understand, the better able you'll be to prepare for your tests, treatment, and appointments with your cardiologist.

With the information in this chapter, you will be more aware of what may be causing your symptoms, when to seek help, and what questions to ask the members of your health-care team. Armed with this knowledge, you should be better able to comprehend your diagnosis, your test results, and your doctor's recommendations.

All this should lead to clearer communication with your doctor, facilitating a better relationship for both of you and resulting in improvement in the quality of your care.

(For detailed descriptions of medications mentioned in this chapter, see Chapter 7.)

DISEASES OF THE AORTA

The aorta is the largest blood vessel in the body. It is the main artery for the entire system of circulation, exiting the heart just above the aortic valve, wrapping around in a "U-turn" within the chest and ending in the pelvic region. From there, the aorta divides into the left and right iliac arteries.

The aorta is divided roughly into several anatomical portions.

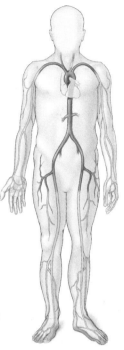

- The *ascending aorta* is the segment within the chest, arising above the aortic valve and extending upward toward the neck.

- The *aortic arch*, also within the chest, is the segment that arches or turns. Major arterial branch vessels arise from the aortic arch, providing blood flow to the head and upper extremities.

- The descending aorta located within the chest cavity is termed the *descending thoracic aorta*.

- Once the descending thoracic aorta passes through the breathing muscle or diaphragm and enters the abdominal cavity, the aorta is termed the *abdominal aorta*.

The circulatory system

Aortic Aneurysm

An aneurysm is a bulging or protrusion of the wall of an artery or the heart. It may be found in any portion of the aorta. In many circumstances, aneurysms are full of atherosclerosis. The atherosclerosis infiltrates and weakens the wall of the artery, causing the aorta to enlarge and eventually bulge. Often, the aorta is found to be enlarged throughout and curving ("ectatic") in its course but without an actual bulge. An ectatic aorta can be a precursor to aneurysm formation.

The risk factors for aneurysm and atherosclerosis formation are similar and include tobacco use, hypertension, and elevated blood lipids. Aggressive prevention of hypertension through diet and exercise, or control of hypertension if blood pressure is already high, may well be the most important intervention to prevent aneurysm formation. Blood-pressure control is important because aneurysms can grow larger with high blood pressure, and large aneurysms can rupture, which can be fatal.

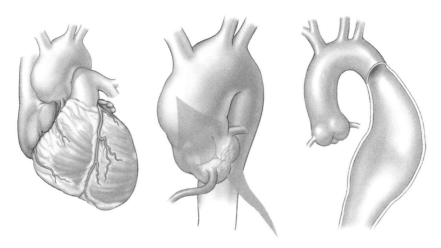

An aneurysm is a bulging or protrusion of the wall of an artery or the heart. It may be found in any portion of the aorta.

Aneurysms without significant atherosclerosis are also possible. Generally there are two causes for aortic aneurysms without atherosclerosis.

- *Untreated high blood pressure,* especially when present for a long time. The elevated blood pressure exerts a significant stress on the wall of the aorta, particularly the ascending aorta.

   This stress results in dilation of the wall and subsequent formation of an aneurysm. In this case, the aneurysm may be located at the level of the aortic valve, causing enlargement of the aortic valve annulus (or ring) and a centrally leaking aortic valve.

- *An intrinsic weakening of the aortic wall itself.* This weakening is believed to be secondary to a structural defect in the connective tissues that comprise the aortic wall. The pathology term for this condition is "cystic medial necrosis." This condition occurs more frequently, but not always, in patients with Marfan's Syndrome.

The symptoms of a thoracic or abdominal aortic aneurysm may include pain that is located in the chest, back, or abdomen.

If an abdominal aortic aneurysm is large enough, the physician can detect it by feeling the abdomen. Other ways of detecting these aneurysms include:

- A routine chest x-ray
- A CT or MRI scan of the chest or abdomen
- An ultrasound examination of the abdominal aorta
- An echocardiogram of the heart

The best tests to uncover the full extent of an aneurysm and to offer precise measurements are the MRI scan and/or the CT scan.

Most aneurysms do not rupture. The likelihood of rupture increases significantly as the aneurysm reaches 5.5 cm in size. In view of these two facts, when you are first diagnosed your doctor may decide on a course of "watchful waiting," rather than recommend surgery on the body's biggest supplier of blood.

The treatment for aortic aneurysm is dictated by the aneurysm's size, location, and rate of growth.

But before the aneurysm can be treated, it is important to normalize your blood pressure and blood lipids through diet, exercise, and medication (if needed). Stopping smoking is imperative. In addition, it is critically important to achieve long-term control of your blood pressure after your aneurysm is repaired.

There are three approaches for the treatment of an aneurysm:

- The first approach is aggressive modification of risk factors such as smoking, high blood pressure, and high blood lipids. The latter two risk factors should be controlled through a combination of lifestyle changes such as a healthy diet (low in sodium and saturated fat) and increased physical activity and medications. This approach is especially important for patients with other medical conditions serious enough to make surgery a significant risk. Risk-factor modification is safe, as patients are not exposed to the risks of invasive procedures.

- The second approach – one that is increasingly employed – is percutaneous endovascular stent graft placement. Endovascular stent grafts represent a medical advance, particularly for those patients who are not candidates for open-chest or abdominal surgery because their level of risk is deemed too high.

In this procedure, a catheter is introduced through the skin in the region of the upper front thigh and is placed spanning the aneurysm. A synthetic, wire-mesh stent graft is then deployed, in effect lining the aneurysm, isolating it, and protecting it from turbulent blood flow. The locations most typically amenable for stent graft use include the abdominal aorta (below the renal arteries) and the descending thoracic aorta. Unfortunately, stent grafts are not suitable for every patient, including those who have aneurysms that span large branching vessels such as the arteries of the kidney.

Stenting requires at least an overnight stay in the hospital to monitor for possible bleeding complications related to the entry point of the catheter.

● The third approach is open surgery. During the operation, the aneurysm is replaced with synthetic tubular graft material. In the case of aneurysms of the ascending aorta and aortic arch, the reparative surgery requires stopping the heart and placing the patient on a heart-lung machine. The aortic valve may be replaced at the same time if it is leaking and cannot be repaired.

Surgery, particularly an operation within the chest cavity, is a high-risk endeavor best carried out only by the most experienced surgeons. This operation is reserved for those patients who have either a large aneurysm or one that is growing (and is thus at high risk of future rupture) and who are otherwise healthy and at low risk of complications from surgery.

Stenting requires at least an overnight stay in the hospital to monitor for possible bleeding complications related to the entry point of the catheter. You may also receive IV medications such as blood-thinners. Before discharge, x-rays are commonly performed to confirm an appropriate and stable stent position. Follow-up testing includes CT scanning and should take place at least yearly.

After open surgery, follow-up CT scans or MRIs will be scheduled. You'll also have your incision followed closely after the operation to make sure that it's healing well.

Aortic Dissection

The aorta has three different cellular layers. An aortic dissection is literally a tear in the aorta, creating a false or additional channel of blood flow within the middle layer of the aorta. An aortic dissection can occur anywhere along the length of the aorta, and it is a true medical emergency.

Most often there are two tears, an entry point through the aorta into the false channel and an exit point from the false channel back into the aorta. The false channel of blood can compress the normal aorta and block or compromise blood flow to vital organs such as the intestines, kidneys, and the lower extremities. The aorta can also "dissect backward," disrupting aortic valve function and causing acute severe valve leakage and congestive heart failure.

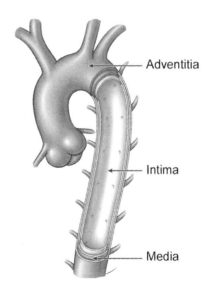

It can also leak blood into the sac around the heart, called the pericardium, creating massive external pressure on the heart chambers. This external pressure can have a negative effect on heart function by markedly reducing the pumping capacity of the heart.

The three different cellular layers of the aorta

Urgent imaging of the aorta is necessary to assess the extent and type of aortic dissection. Imaging can take three forms: transesophageal echocardiography (TEE), CT, or MRI. TEE involves the passage of a small flexible tube, similar to an endoscope, through the mouth to the esophagus. An ultrasound crystal on the end of the probe permits the physician to visualize the heart and its surrounding structures. (CT and MRI are explained in detail in Chapter 5.) The construction of a management plan will be based on the results of the imaging study.

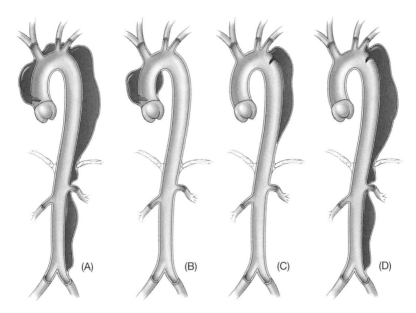

Aortic dissection. *Blood has dissected within the inner layers of the aorta (shaded areas), creating a false channel (A) throughout the entire aortic length, (B) confined to the ascending aorta just above the aortic valve, (C) confined to the descending thoracic aorta, (D) confined to the descending thoracic and abdominal aorta.*

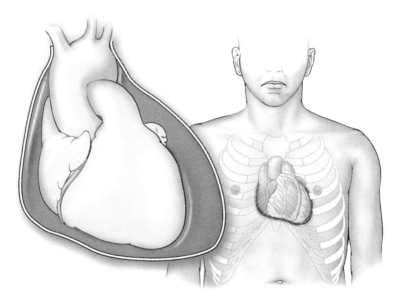

Pericardial effusion. *A potential complication of aortic dissection whereby blood collects within the pericardial sac, in advanced cases compressing the exterior of the heart and compromising the heart's output of blood.*

Not all aortic dissections require surgery. Some will heal spontaneously, particularly when blood pressure is lowered and stabilized. The location of the aortic tear and the degree to which blood flow to vital organs is compromised will determine which approach is pursued: "watchful waiting" or surgery.

Aortic Stenosis

The aortic valve is one of heart's four valves. These valves direct blood flow within the heart, maintaining efficient transport of oxygen to the body's vital organs and tissues. The aortic valve is uniquely positioned on the oxygen-rich left side of the heart, situated between the left ventricle (the main pumping chamber of the heart) and the aorta (the main blood vessel exiting the heart). The aortic valve has three thin leaflets that open and close approximately 100,000 times per day.

Under normal circumstances, the aortic valve opens fully while the heart is pumping, a process known as systole. Between heartbeats (during cardiac relaxation), the aortic valve closes fully. This is known as diastole.

In aortic stenosis, the aortic valve leaflets don't fully open during cardiac systole. The restricted leaflet opening impedes the flow of blood

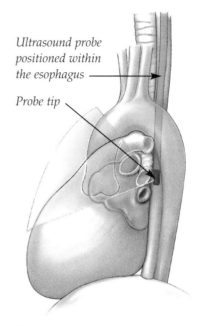

Ultrasound probe positioned within the esophagus

Probe tip

Physicians can visualize the heart during TEE imaging.

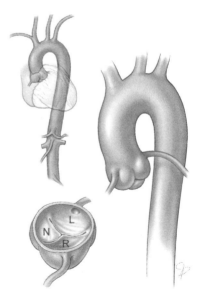

The aortic valve has three thin leaflets that open and close approximately 100,000 times per day.

from the left ventricle to the aorta. This impediment to blood flow creates a pressure difference across the aortic valve between the left ventricle and aorta. The left ventricle must then generate greater pressure to maintain an effective flow of blood (known as the "cardiac output") across the restricted opening of the aortic valve.

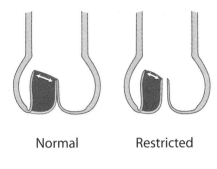

Normal   Restricted

In aortic stenosis, the aortic valve leaflets don't fully open during cardiac systole.

In advanced cases of aortic stenosis, the pressure required to maintain sufficient circulatory blood flow produces inordinate strain on the left ventricle. This increased strain results in thickening of the heart muscle, a condition termed "left ventricular hypertrophy." If aortic stenosis is left untreated, progressive thickening of the left ventricle ensues, followed by enlargement of the left ventricle and irreversible weakening of the heart muscle.

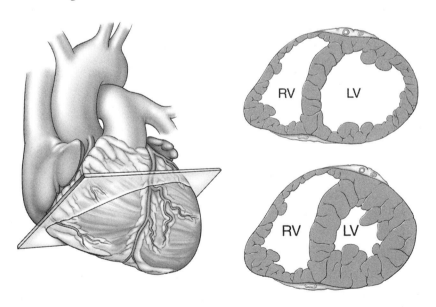

Increased left ventricular strain results in a thickening of the heart muscle (termed "left ventricular hypertrophy").

The causes of aortic stenosis include:

- Congenitally abnormal aortic valves may cause aortic stenosis, with symptoms beginning in a patient's 30s or 40s.
- Acute rheumatic fever, a streptococcus infection that occurs most often during childhood, may result in the appearance of aortic stenosis decades later.
- Most commonly, aortic stenosis results from a progressive thickening and degenerative process of the aortic valve and usually manifests anywhere from age 60 to 90.

The most effective treatment for symptomatic aortic stenosis is surgical replacement of the aortic valve. The three classic symptoms of advanced aortic stenosis are angina pectoris (cardiac discomfort in the chest), pre-syncope or syncope (near-fainting or fainting), and CHF.

Aortic Insufficiency

Aortic insufficiency is a form of valvular heart disease in which the aortic valve leaflets fail to close fully ("coapt") during relaxation ("ventricular diastole"). This failure to coapt results in the backward flow of oxygenated blood from the ascending aorta to the left ventricle. This is a highly inefficient and abnormal development as a portion of the oxygenated blood is no longer propelled forward. In addition, the left ventricular chamber is subject to an increasing volume of blood, which raises pressures within the heart and stresses the left ventricular heart wall.

In advanced and longstanding cases of aortic valve insufficiency, the heart begins to enlarge (dilate) and weaken, reducing its pumping capacity. Congestive heart failure may develop along with pulmonary congestion (fluid retention in the lungs), an ominous sign.

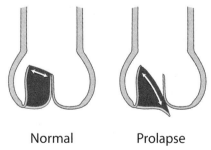

Normal   Prolapse

With aortic insufficiency, the aortic valve leaflets fail to come together fully.

Echocardiography is used to assess aortic insufficiency. If the condition is moderately severe to severe, the best treatment is open-heart surgery and aortic valve replacement before heart function is compromised and congestive heart failure develops.

The risks of valve replacement include stroke, heart attack, kidney dysfunction, infection, and death, although, as with other cardiac operations, these risks diminish significantly when the procedure is performed in carefully selected patients by an experienced surgeon.

Follow-up to surgery should include a four- to six-week postoperative checkup and yearly echocardiograms.

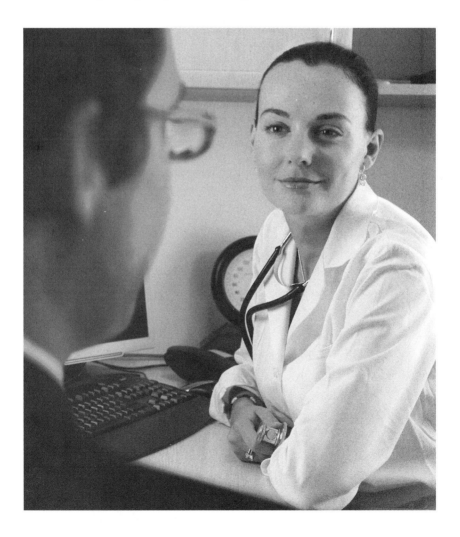

Any weakening of the heart muscle and enlargement of the heart may be irreversible, even after valve-replacement surgery. So it's extremely important to report any symptoms of CHF, including:

- Shortness of breath during rest or upon exertion
- Unexplained weight gain (most likely retained fluid)
- Swelling in the lower extremities

ANGINA PECTORIS (CHEST PAIN)

Angina pectoris (cardiac chest discomfort or pain) is a long-recognized symptom of coronary artery obstruction. It manifests when coronary artery blockages limit blood flow and oxygen delivery to the heart muscle, and therefore the reduced oxygen supply is unable to meet the requisite oxygen demand.

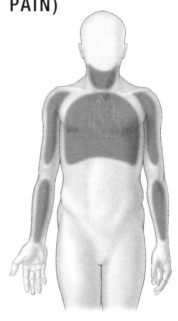

Most often, patients describe a chest pressure or discomfort centrally located below the breastbone (sternum), with a greater predilection for the left side of the chest (but not always). The discomfort is generally within a region of the chest described as the size of a clenched fist.

The discomfort of angina pectoris may travel or radiate to the throat, neck, jaw, teeth, or arms.

The discomfort may travel or radiate to the throat, neck, jaw, teeth, or arms. Should the discomfort radiate to the arms, there is a greater tendency for angina pectoris to be experienced in the left arm.

In most circumstances, angina pectoris occurs during periods of physical exertion when the heart muscle's oxygen requirements are high. As obstruction of the coronary artery progresses, however, less and less activity is required to provoke symptoms. In extreme cases, you may experience angina pectoris with minimal or no activity.

When angina pectoris is in its early phase (provoked by activity and ceasing with rest), you may find yourself unconsciously adjusting your activity patterns, such as walking at a slower pace or taking the elevator instead of stairs, in an effort to reduce or avoid symptoms. Although this is a good idea, it should not replace seeking immediate medical attention.

If you have angina that is considered stable – that is, it's predictable, mild, and resolves when you stop your activity – your physician may recommend a trial of medications. This trial may last several months to gauge the effects of the medications being used.

Typically, the medications prescribed aim to reduce blood pressure and pulse rate, which lowers the heart muscle's demand for oxygen. In addition, there are other medications that directly dilate (enlarge) the coronary arteries, increasing the amount of oxygen delivered to the heart muscle.

These medications improve symptoms but have only a temporary effect. This is because even though they either increase the supply of oxygen or reduce the demand for it – and thereby reduce the frequency and/or severity of the angina episodes – they don't affect the root cause of the problem: the atherosclerosis.

That's why your doctor may recommend a heart catheterization. A catheterization will clearly delineate the number and severity of any heart blockages, and permit the development of the best therapeutic plan. That being said, it is totally reasonable to try an initial course of medication in stable angina patients.

It's important to understand that the obstruction that is causing your angina symptoms is not necessarily the basis for a future heart attack. Other obstructions or atherosclerotic plaques that haven't caused angina may acutely rupture and cause a heart attack. At the present time, it is not possible to identify which atherosclerotic plaque is the most likely to rupture. This is an important scientific and clinical challenge that has yet to be solved. Interestingly, while angioplasty and stenting of coronary atherosclerotic obstructions have been proven to relieve symptoms, they have not been shown to prevent future heart attacks or extend life.

Stents are therefore usually reserved for those patients whose angina does not go away when they stop their activity or whose angina is getting worse, which is termed accelerating or "unstable" angina.

If you suspect that you may have angina pectoris, seek medical attention immediately. Also, if you notice that your angina changes pattern (occurs more often, lasts much longer, or is more severe), call your physician. A heart catheterization or other tests may be needed.

ATRIAL FIBRILLATION (AF, AFIB)

Atrial fibrillation is an aberrant cardiac rhythm that affects approximately 10 percent of people age 80 or older. Normally, the upper chambers of the heart, known as the atria, beat in a synchronized manner with the lower chambers, the ventricles. The heart's natural or intrinsic cardiac pacemaker, located in the upper right cardiac chamber, dictates this synchronized beating or contraction. This pacemaker is known as the sinus node.

When Afib is present, instead of the sinus node discharging at a regular normal rate between 60 and 100 times per minute, the atrial electrical impulses discharge in a chaotic and disorganized manner, at a rate between 400 and 600 times per minute.

About 25 percent of these atrial electrical impulses reach the ventricles by way of the AV (atrioventricular) node. The uncoordinated contraction pattern of the atria results in inefficient cardiac function, reducing cardiac output and thus reducing effective blood flow. Additionally, the inefficiency often creates currents of swirling atrial blood in which a blood clot (thrombus) may form. If a clot occurs, it can sometimes travel (embolize) to the brain and cause a stroke.

An effective treatment for Afib is a procedure termed "direct current cardioversion" (DCC). In DCC, you are sedated and rendered unconscious with a short-acting IV anesthetic. Two paddles are applied to your chest, and your heart is briefly subjected to an electric shock. This resets the natural pacemaker of the heart and restores a normal rhythm. To maintain normalcy, many patients remain on cardiac medications after successful DCC.

An alternate strategy is to administer medications that assist in restoring the normal heart rhythm, along with blood-thinners to prevent clotting. Each situation is individualized and best left to a detailed discussion between patient and physician.

Sometimes, both medication and cardioversion are necessary. Medications can both raise the likelihood of cardioversion success and assist in maintaining a normal heart rhythm after cardioversion.

If you are going to have DCC, it's likely that you'll be prescribed the blood-thinner warfarin for three weeks before your procedure. This is to reduce the risk of clot formation.

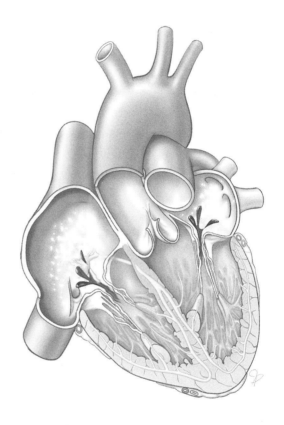

When atrial fibrillation is present, instead of the sinus node discharging at a regular normal rate between 60 and 100 times per minute, the atrial electrical impulses (indicated by the arrows above) discharge in a chaotic and disorganized manner, at a rate between 400 and 600 times per minute.

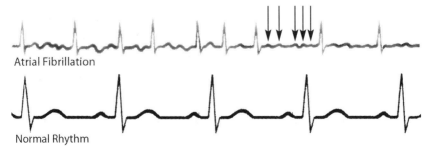

Atrial Fibrillation

Normal Rhythm

However, TEE (transesophageal echocardiography) is being used increasingly to determine whether the usual three weeks of anticoagulation can be avoided before the cardioversion. (See page 82 for a description of TEE.) If TEE shows that conditions do not favor clot formation, and especially if no clot is seen, you can proceed directly to cardioversion.

After a successful cardioversion, anticoagulation with warfarin is continued for a minimum of four more weeks. This is because even though the electrical function of the atria returns to normal following the cardioversion, the *mechanical* function lags behind. The atria don't pump in their normal manner right after a cardioversion because they are stunned and weakened by the atrial fibrillation. Therefore, it's still possible for a clot to form and be dislodged. It takes approximately four weeks for mechanical function of the atria to return to normal.

If you have a high likelihood of atrial fibrillation recurrence, as in patients with mitral stenosis, warfarin may be continued long term.

Should the atrial fibrillation be permanent, oral anticoagulants may be needed indefinitely.

As an alternative to DCC and antiarrhythmic medication, an emerging treatment for Afib is radiofrequency ablation (RFA). This procedure involves passing a number of carefully placed catheters with recording electrodes attached (by means of the blood vessels) to both the upper and lower cardiac chambers. Under x-ray guidance, radiofrequency energy is delivered to precise sites within the heart to permanently ablate (interrupt) the locations where Afib originates.

The risks with radiofrequency ablation are the same as those for any catheter procedure: blood-vessel injury, infection, and the risk (extremely rare) of puncturing the heart. Another risk unique to ablation is pulmonary vein stenosis, in which scarring from the ablation procedure results in a narrowing of the pulmonary veins as they enter the atria. Patients routinely undergo CT scanning of the heart within the first six months after the procedure to evaluate for this possibility.

If you undergo RFA, it is important to take your medications as prescribed, including anticoagulants. In addition, you should be vigilant about noting any symptoms that are related to abnormal heartbeats, such as lightheadedness or near-fainting. Even though radiofrequency ablation cures a high percentage of patients, a small percentage will experience a recurrence of arrhythmia.

ATRIAL FLUTTER

Similar to atrial fibrillation, atrial flutter represents an abnormal heart rhythm emanating from one of the upper cardiac chambers (atria). Robert – remember Robert from the first chapter? – had atrial flutter.

This disturbance of cardiac rhythm can result in extremely rapid ventricular (lower chamber) heart rates, reducing the amount of blood filling the lower ventricular chamber and thus reducing the heart's output of blood. Causes of atrial flutter are numerous and similar to those of atrial fibrillation. Some of the more prominent ones are:

- Valvular heart disease
- Coronary artery disease
- Past or present heart attack
- An overactive thyroid gland
- Chronic lung disease
- Anemia
- Hypertension and resultant heart-muscle thickening
- Unremitting pericarditis

Treatment for atrial flutter is initially focused on slowing the heart rate with a combination of oral and IV medications (given for about one to two days). Slowing the heart rate enables the heart to fill with blood more effectively during the relaxation phase and positively influences the output of blood from the heart.

In the minority of cases, medications will spontaneously convert atrial flutter to normal sinus rhythm, but most patients undergo direct current cardioversion, as described above.

In situations in which atrial flutter is recurrent despite the best combination of medications, radiofrequency ablation is a viable option.

Why Robert Had Atrial Fibrillation

Since one of the possible causes of atrial flutter is an overactive thyroid gland, Dr. Smith decided to order a few thyroid blood tests for Robert. The results were, in fact, consistent with an overactive thyroid.

When questioned, Robert mentioned other things he'd noticed over the previous few months, not realizing they were symptoms of a health problem. He'd had an unexplained 10-pound weight loss, a constant jittery or "wired" feeling, and an elevation of his resting heart rate. And he always felt warm, even in air-conditioned rooms. Putting all this together in retrospect made the diagnosis quite clear.

Fortunately for Robert, his atrial flutter was not due to a primary cardiac cause but was instead secondary to his abnormally functioning thyroid gland. Nonetheless, he needed to have the atrial flutter treated.

In addition to warfarin, Dr. Smith prescribed a beta blocker, metoprolol, at a dose of 25 mg, twice daily. Dr. Smith referred Robert to an endocrinologist (a thyroid specialist), and Robert received prompt, effective treatment for his overactive thyroid.

Within a few months Robert noted a reduction, and later the elimination, of all symptoms. Dr. Smith was able to safely discontinue both the warfarin and metoprolol.

ATRIAL TACHYCARDIA

A heart-rhythm disturbance similar to atrial flutter, atrial tachycardia originates from a single atrial location. The medications and procedures used to treat atrial tachycardia are nearly identical with those used for atrial flutter.

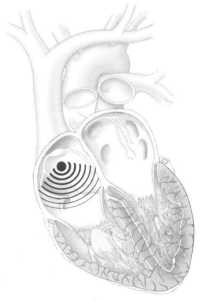

Atrial tachycardia is a heart-rhythm disturbance that originates from a single atrial location.

BACTERIAL INFECTIVE ENDOCARDITIS

Infrequently, the heart can be subject to a bacterial infection. Bacteria enter the bloodstream on a regular basis, especially when you brush your teeth. The bacteria are normally "filtered" without consequence by the immune system and circulating infection-fighting cells.

When a patient has abnormal heart valves, particularly valves that are degenerative and thickened, circulating bacteria can "stick" to the irregular valve surfaces. Without prompt and appropriate antibiotic treatment, bacteria that adhere to the valve surfaces can multiply. This is called "bacterial endocarditis." A common cause of bacterial endo-carditis is poor dental hygiene combined with vigorous dental cleaning.

Once a critical mass of bacteria is reached, valve destruction ensues, eroding valve tissue. The damaged valve tissue renders the valve incompetent or regurgitant (leaking) – often severely so.

Endocarditis is diagnosed by drawing blood, growing the bacteria in the microbiology laboratory, and observing infected valve tissue on an echocardiogram. Treatment is with antibiotics for a minimum of four to six weeks.

Following antibiotic therapy, you will need an echocardiogram to reestablish your new baseline value function, plus close follow-up with echocardiograms, which are typically performed at 6- and 12-month intervals. Your physician will also want to listen to your heart periodically to assess the function of your valve.

Not all patients diagnosed with bacterial infective endocarditis suf-fer severe valve damage. In fact, if diagnosed early, endocarditis can be cured solely with antibiotics, with minimal residual valve damage.

Patients who have severe valve disease as a result of endocarditis need valve repair or replacement surgery. Treating the infection com-pletely before proceeding with valve surgery is the preferred approach because an ongoing infection at the time of valve surgery increases the risk of infecting the new valve. Waiting to do surgery may not be an option when endocarditis is present, however, because of the risk of complications such as abscess formation, congestive heart failure, and persistent signs of infection despite high-dose IV antibiotics.

If you have been diagnosed with bacterial infective endocarditis, you will probably need to take antibiotics before any medical or dental procedures, and you must practice good dental and personal hygiene in order to reduce the risk of infecting the valve again.

The American Heart Association issues a convenient wallet-sized card concisely outlining current recommendations for endocarditis prophylaxis. These guidelines have recently been updated. It is also readily available on the Internet at http://www.americanheart.org (at the web page, search for "endocarditis prophylaxis").

BRADY-TACHY SYNDROME

Aging can slow the normal transmission of the heart's electrical impulses. This slowing can also be associated with a malfunctioning sinus node, the collection of nerve fibers that serves as the heart's pacemaker.

A malfunctioning sinus node can cause (and propagate) the heart's electrical impulses to be discharged in a disorderly fashion, intermittently creating both abnormally slow and fast heartbeats in an unpredictable manner. You may feel your heart beating rapidly with intermittent episodes of lightheadedness and near-fainting, reflecting both the fast and slow heartbeats.

You may feel your heart beating rapidly with intermittent episodes of lightheadedness and near-fainting, reflecting both the fast and slow heartbeats.

Treating brady-tachy syndrome is challenging. Taking medications to treat the intermittent fast heartbeats causes even slower heart rates, exacerbating symptoms of lightheadedness and fainting.

When they are symptomatic, patients with brady-tachy syndrome are best treated by implantation of a permanent pacemaker. A pacemaker permits medicines to be given to treat the rapid heartbeats while at the same time providing a steady backup heart rate, thereby preventing untoward slowing of your pulse. In fact, the brady-tachy syndrome is one of the most common indications for permanent pacemaker placement.

WHAT IS A PACEMAKER, AND FOR WHAT OTHER DISEASES IS IT USED?

A cardiac pacemaker consists of two components, the pulse generator and the pacemaker leads. Over the years, these devices have become more sophisticated while becoming much smaller. The pulse generator is the power source. It also contains complex computerized circuitry that is individually programmed to the specific needs and activity level of the patient.

Pacemakers are implanted when patients experience – or are at risk for – a severe slowing of their heart rate. The most common cause of a slowed heart rate is the primary degeneration of the heart's conduction system, as with aging. This degenerative process can culminate in a condition known as "conduction block," in which the electrical impulse originating from the

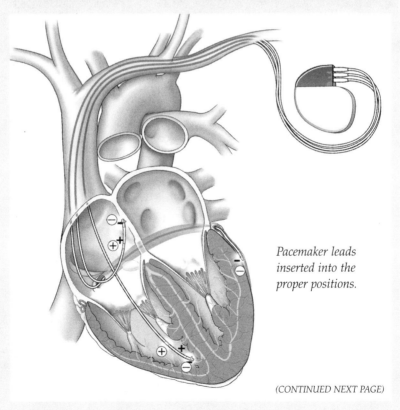

Pacemaker leads inserted into the proper positions.

(CONTINUED NEXT PAGE)

top chamber of the heart is prevented from transmitting to the bottom chamber. This causes slow backup or "escape" rhythms, which the patient feels as profound fatigue or lassitude.

The placement of a cardiac pacemaker most often requires an overnight hospital stay. Similar to an implantable cardiac defibrillator, a small, shallow incision about 2 inches long is made below the collarbone, and a pocket is constructed under the skin. The pulse generator is positioned within the pocket once the pacemaker leads are in proper position. The pacemaker leads are inserted through a large vein, generally the left subclavian vein. Under x-ray guidance, the lead tips are precisely positioned within the right ventricular cardiac apex (tip) and the right atrial appendage (a small outpouching of right atrial tissue through which blood enters and exits, something like a dead-end street). The leads are subsequently attached to the pulse generator and the pacemaker's pocket incision is sutured closed.

There are few risks to pacemaker insertion. They include infection of the pacemaker pocket, infection of the leads, damage to the tricuspid (right-sided) valve, perforation of the heart, blood-vessel damage, and a punctured lung. Despite these potentially serious complications, pacemakers are implanted daily and the small, cumulative risk of insertion is far outweighed by the benefit conferred.

Pacemakers are complex devices that are programmed by a computer. The device is routinely checked for proper functioning and battery life over the phone and in person. Most pacemakers, depending upon their level of use, are replaced within 10 years of initial placement. If functioning well, the leads will remain in place, simplifying the repeat procedure.

An important feature of current pacemakers is called "rate responsivity." Under normal circumstances, with increased activity and therefore increased demands by the body for oxygen, the heart rate increases proportionately. Rate responsivity allows the pacemaker to simulate the body's normal response of increased heart rate by monitoring body motion or respiratory rate. Rate responsivity permits patients to continue to enjoy a normally active lifestyle without significant heart rate limitation.

CAROTID ATHEROSCLEROSIS

Carotid atherosclerosis is the same process that commonly affects the coronary arteries, but it is located within the carotid (neck) arteries. The carotid arteries are the major conduits for delivering oxygen-rich blood to the brain. Patients with carotid artery disease are at risk for stroke and therefore merit careful monitoring.

Carotid artery atherosclerosis is common in persons who have atherosclerotic disease in the coronary arteries, aorta, and arteries of the lower extremities.

An examination of the carotid arteries is an important part of a complete physical examination. The physician typically listens over the anterolateral (at the front and slightly to each side) aspects of the

Patients with carotid artery disease are at risk for stroke and therefore merit careful monitoring.

neck, over the carotid pulse. A whooshing sound (called a "bruit") typically indicates an obstruction of the carotid artery.

Although the carotid artery has narrowed, the same amount of blood must pass through it to deliver oxygen to the brain. When significant narrowing is present, the blood is "forced" across the blockage and the velocity of blood flow increases. A "spray jet" of turbulence results; this is what is heard as a bruit.

Additionally, the physician may feel (palpate) your carotid pulse to assess its intensity or strength. Using gentle pressure, he may compare the intensity of the left and right carotid pulses simultaneously. This technique permits a qualitative assessment of pulse intensity. Reduced pulse strength can serve as the first clinical clue to carotid atherosclerosis.

Carotid vascular ultrasound has proven to be an outstanding tool to assess and follow a patient with carotid atherosclerosis. It is entirely painless and without known risk.

The procedure uses technology identical to that of a cardiac ultrasound (echocardiogram), but in this instance, the ultrasound transducer is placed on your neck to transmit images of the carotid arteries and blood flow through these arteries.

Measuring the velocity of blood flow and comparing it to established norms permits an accurate estimate of the severity of the blockage. If the blockage is not severe, you will be followed on a regular basis, generally annually. If the blockage obstructs 80 percent to 99 percent of the artery, the risk of stroke increases significantly and a reparative procedure is recommended.

SURGERY OR STENT?

The treatment of carotid artery disease continues to evolve. In the past, open surgery was recommended in which the carotid artery was directly visualized and the atherosclerotic debris was removed. This is termed a "carotid endarterectomy." This procedure can carry a high risk, especially for patients who have other significant illnesses, such as advanced coronary artery disease and/or congestive heart failure.

Now, carotid artery stents similar to those made for coronary arteries have been developed. The stent, a meshlike structure, is deployed through a catheter and, once deployed, buttresses the atherosclerotic debris against the artery wall, greatly improving blood flow.

A concern with stenting of carotid arteries is the risk of atherosclerotic plaque breaking off during the procedure and then traveling to and lodging within the brain, resulting in a stroke. Innovative devices (called "embolic protection devices") are now routinely used during the procedure to significantly reduce this likelihood. When deployed within the carotid artery, these devices resemble an open umbrella, catching the dislodged atherosclerotic pieces of plaque and reducing the chance of a stroke.

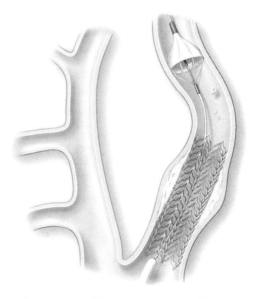

The stent, a meshlike structure, resembles an umbrella within the carotid artery.

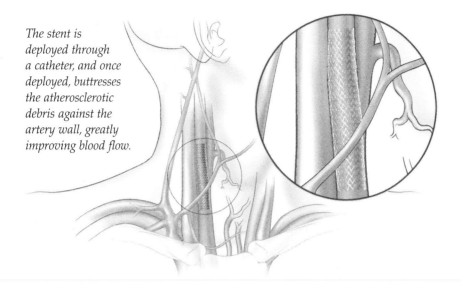

The stent is deployed through a catheter, and once deployed, buttresses the atherosclerotic debris against the artery wall, greatly improving blood flow.

The choice of a carotid artery stent versus a carotid endarterectomy is best made through a careful consultation with your physician. The location of the obstruction may be a factor. Also, other preexisting medical conditions may make open carotid surgery too risky, thus making a carotid stent a safer option. The risk with carotid endarterectomy in a patient with other medical conditions lies not in the operation itself but in the need for general anesthesia, which is not as safe, for example, in a person with active congestive heart failure, accelerating or unstable angina, severe uncontrolled hypertension, or a recent heart attack.

CLAUDICATION

Claudication is a symptom of lower extremity (leg) atherosclerosis and compromised blood flow to the muscles. It is described most frequently as a burning sensation felt in one or both calves, especially when the patient is walking. It can also be located in the buttocks. Where the sensations occur depends upon the site(s) of the arterial blockage.

Claudication symptoms reflect inadequate blood supply to skeletal muscle. This inadequate supply occurs most often during periods of increased activity (and therefore higher oxygen demand). If you experience claudication symptoms, the likelihood of narrowing in arteries of the lower extremities is high. If left untreated, claudication in extreme circumstances can result in gangrenous tissue and the need for amputation. In addition, given the poor oxygen delivery to the feet and toes, healing of wounds in these areas might be delayed or, in the worst case, these wounds may not heal at all, leading to infection and possibly amputation, especially if infection spreads to the bone (osteomyelitis).

An angiogram can locate the presence and extent of narrowing in the lower extremities. Once the area of narrowing is defined, angioplasty and stenting, or surgical bypass, can restore adequate blood flow to the legs just as atherosclerosis is treated in the heart.

Medications also exist that will improve symptoms, but typically they will not restore normal function completely. One such medication is called cilostazol, which helps dilate the arteries and improve blood flow. Cilostazol neither speeds healing of wounds nor reduces risk of infection, but it may improve quality of life. (This medication cannot be used if you have a history of congestive heart failure.)

Claudication can be the first clue to the presence of atherosclerosis in other arteries. Once it is diagnosed, your physician must search for atherosclerosis in other areas, including the carotid and coronary arteries. This further investigation may entail a carotid artery ultrasound and a stress test.

CONGESTIVE HEART FAILURE (CHF): TWO MAIN TYPES

Systolic Heart Failure

The main cause of CHF is a weakening of the heart's left ventricle, which causes it to pump blood out of the heart ineffectively. CHF due to heart-muscle weakening is termed "systolic heart failure."

Reduction of forward blood flow with systolic heart failure results in delivery of an inadequate supply of oxygen to the tissues and can compromise the function of organs, including the kidneys.

The reduced blood flow can also increase the volume of blood and pressure in the heart, thereby increasing the workload of the heart. When chronic, this increased heart stress can result in further deterioration of heart function.

Untreated congestive heart failure passes through predictable stages of increasing severity. Daily activities become more severely impaired with each stage.

The increased volume of blood and pressure in the heart is transmitted "backward" to the lungs, causing lung congestion, increased lung pressures, and breathlessness. In advanced cases, the increased lung pressure (pulmonary hypertension) is irreversible. In such cases, fluid accumulates in the abdomen and intractable swelling occurs in the lower extremities. When this happens, the risk of death is high.

Diastolic Heart Failure

Another form of CHF, one that is recognized increasingly, is termed "diastolic heart failure." This is a failure of the heart's left ventricle to relax properly. It is typically seen with longstanding high blood pressure and at least moderate thickening of the walls of the left ventricle of the heart.

It is typically seen with longstanding high blood pressure and at least moderate thickening of the walls of the left ventricle of the heart.

With diastolic heart failure, pressures within the heart increase for any given volume of blood. This phenomenon occurs because the heart's walls are less compliant.

For example, if 50 cc of fluid are present in the left ventricle, the pressure will increase only slightly if the ventricle is compliant. In contrast, if the left ventricle is stiff, the pressure will rise much more. Therefore, with diastolic heart failure, the heart muscle is much less forgiving and does not relax as well for any given amount of fluid. In fact, during a period of exceptionally high blood pressure, a temporary disturbance of the heart rhythm, or high salt consumption, blood volume and pressure within the heart may rise to a critical level to cause fluid to accumulate in the lungs.

The most common symptom experienced in both types of heart failure is shortness of breath during exertion. Diastolic heart failure can be attenuated by reversing its underlying cause, whether it is high blood pressure, an abnormal heart rhythm, or use of too much salt.

TREATMENT
Treatment of congestive heart failure is best directed at both the underlying cause and symptom relief. In patients with hypertension, normalization of blood pressure is imperative. In patients with coronary artery disease and weakened heart muscle, improving coronary circulation by means of angioplasty, stent, or bypass surgery can improve the strength of the heart muscle.

Dual chamber defibrillators (biventricular implantable defibrillators, or Bi-V ICDs) can help synchronize left and right ventricular function and improve symptoms.

Medications typically employed include beta blockers, ACE inhibitors, and diuretics.

DILATED CARDIOMYOPATHY

Dilated cardiomyopathy is another condition in which the heart muscle becomes weakened. Because the muscle is weak, the heart can't pump sufficient blood out of the ventricle, so a greater volume remains behind after each heartbeat. As the ventricle retains more and more blood, it gets bigger, eventually causing the muscle walls to become even weaker. This can lead to progressive congestive heart failure.

The most common cause of dilated cardiomyopathy is a virus, such as those responsible for the common cold. For reasons that are inexplicable and fortunately rare, the virus exerts an inflammatory effect on the heart muscle, irreparably damaging its fibers. This condition, which can lead to dilated cardiomyopathy, is called "myocarditis."

Other causes of cardiomyopathy are:

- Toxins, such as excessive alcohol ingested over a long period of time or environmental toxins such as lead and mercury

- Longstanding anemia, such as sickle cell disease, that overworks the heart
- Profound thyroid disorders
- Pregnancy (albeit rare)
- Some medications, such as a select group of chemotherapeutic agents

The treatment of dilated cardiomyopathy depends on the cause and the severity of the heart's dysfunction.

- In the best-case scenario, the heart muscle is initially inflamed, but the underlying condition either abates (in the case of a virus) or is successfully treated (such as happens with thyroid disorders) and the heart returns to normal function.
- In intermediate cases, the cause (for example, excessive alcohol use) is eliminated or rectified and the heart muscle improves, although it does not return to its normal function. In this situation, the patient may or may not develop symptoms of CHF, which depends on the level of remaining heart function.
- In advanced cases, which represent the minority of cardiomyopathy patients, the heart muscle is severely weakened and the patient experiences profound CHF and must be placed on the cardiac transplantation waiting list for a new heart.

Except for those who completely recover heart-muscle function, patients are prescribed medication aimed at reducing the work of the heart by lowering the blood pressure and pulse rate. Often, when the symptoms of CHF are caused by cardiomyopathy, they can be controlled with medication, and quality of life is close to normal.

HEART MURMUR

A heart murmur is a heart sound the doctor can hear with a stethoscope. The classical heart murmurs originate from abnormal heart valves. When the heart's valves do not open fully (stenosis) or do not close fully (leak or regurgitate), your physician will hear abnormal sounds. Depending upon the valve and their cause, these sounds are located in specific areas of the chest wall and their timing is predictable in relation to the pulse.

Heart murmurs are not always loud, and detecting them may depend on the experience and meticulousness of the listening physician. In particular, faint diastolic murmurs can be overlooked during a cursory examination.

Heart Murmur

Normal

Under normal circumstances, valve leaflets open fully, directing an unimpeded flow of blood, and close completely, without observed blood leakage.

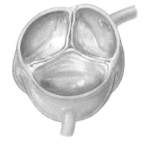
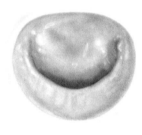

Leaky (prolapsed)

In a prolapsed valve, one or more valve leaflets do not completely coapt (close together). Depending upon the degree of coaptation, the result is mild, moderate, or severe valve leakage.

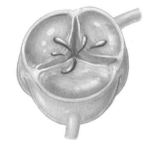
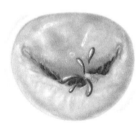

Stenotic (restricted)

A stenotic valve does not open fully. This renders a heightened pressure difference (transvalvular gradient) across the valve and increases the work of the heart.

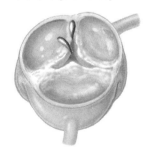
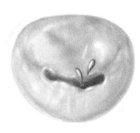

Once a heart murmur is identified, the physician must evaluate its location, timing, and intensity to decide whether it is an "innocent" or a pathological finding. If your doctor suspects the murmur is problematic, his next step will be to order an echocardiogram to determine its presence and severity.

In conjunction with measurements of heart size and function, the echocardiogram guides the treatment strategy. If the valve abnormality is found to be mild, no follow-up other than periodic heart examinations is warranted. If it is more severe, you will need more frequent physician visits, including regular examinations and echocardiograms performed about once a year.

Heart murmurs can occur under expected circumstances as in childhood, during pregnancy, or in the presence of anemia. But heart murmurs can also indicate serious structural heart disease. It is your doctor's task to differentiate between innocent and serious heart murmurs.

HEART BLOCK

The heart's electrical system can short-circuit either temporarily or permanently. Heart block represents a block in the electrical impulse that travels from the upper cardiac chambers (atria) to the lower cardiac chambers (ventricles). The most common cause of heart block is degenerative aging of the heart's electrical conduction system.

Initially, the electrical impulses are slowed and appear on the electrocardiogram as "prolonged conduction intervals." This means that it is taking longer for each electrical impulse to travel within the heart and arrive at its destination. The heart rate also slows. These slowed conduction intervals can lead to intermittent blocked or nonconducted electrical impulses that fail to reach the ventricles, causing the heart's pumping to be delayed.

In advanced cases, heart block can reduce the heart's output of blood and reduce blood flow to the brain, causing transient lightheadedness, near-fainting, or even fainting. When the symptoms of heart block are persistent, implantation of a permanent pacemaker is indicated.

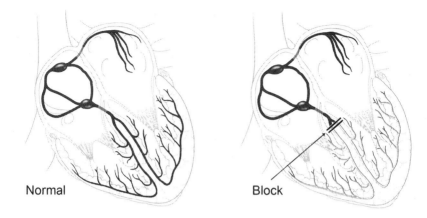

Normal   Block

Heart block represents a block in the electrical impulse that travels from the upper cardiac chambers (atria) to the lower cardiac chambers (ventricles).

In addition to aging, other causes of heart block include certain medications that slow cardiac conduction (beta blockers and calcium channel blockers); impaired blood flow from the coronary arteries to the conduction system tissue, causing the conduction system to function abnormally; and certain diseases that infiltrate the heart and damage the conduction system (for example, sarcoidosis). With these conditions, heart block may be transient or persistent, often treated with a permanent pacemaker.

HYPERLIPIDEMIA

Hyperlipidemia is a condition in which a person has high levels of one or more components of lipids (fats) in the bloodstream. These components include cholesterol (predominantly "bad" LDL and "good" HDL) and triglycerides.

High levels of blood fats are a risk factor for atherosclerosis and potential heart attack.

In 2003, a new set of cholesterol guidelines was issued for both health-care professionals and patients in which optimal, normal, and high levels of certain lipids were defined.

According to these guidelines, all adults at least 20 years old should have a lipoprotein profile (blood test) performed after fasting.

If normal, this should be repeated at a minimum of every five years. This profile includes a measurement of serum total cholesterol, LDL cholesterol, HDL cholesterol, and triglyceride (blood fat) levels.

If your levels are not optimal, first-line treatment is to eat a low-fat diet, exercise regularly, attain an ideal body weight, normalize blood pressure, and avoid tobacco. Medication may also be added if your levels are still too high.

Lipid-lowering medications, also known as cholesterol-lowering medications, have been proven in large research trials to reduce the risk of death, heart attacks, and other cardiac events in people who are at risk for (e.g. diabetics) or have documented atherosclerosis.

Patients at high risk for atherosclerosis, such as those with diabetes or high blood pressure, smokers, and those with a strong family history of coronary artery disease, have also been shown to benefit from cholesterol-lowering medications. In fact, those patients with documented coronary artery disease have even more aggressive LDL lowering goals with a target level of less than or equal to 70 mg/dl.

CHOLESTEROL GUIDELINES		
LDL Cholesterol	<100 mg/dL	Optimal
	100-129 mg/dL	Near optimal/above optimal
	130-159 mg/dL	Borderline high
	160-189 mg/dL	High
	≥190 mg/dL	Very high
Total Cholesterol	<200 mg/dL	Desirable
	200-239 mg/dL	Borderline High
	≥240 mg/dL	High
HDL Cholesterol	<40 mg/dL	Low (not preferred)
	≥60 mg/dL	High (preferred)

http://www.nhlbi.nih.gov/guidelines/cholesterol/atp3xsum.pdf

Epidemiologists have studied the association between lipid levels and events related to coronary heart disease. They found that for each 1 percent reduction in LDL cholesterol levels, the risk of a heart attack or death related to coronary heart disease also drops by 1 percent. The association between HDL cholesterol and cardiac events is even stronger: Each 1 percent increase in HDL cholesterol decreases the risk of cardiac events by 2 percent to 3 percent.

For details on lipid-lowering medications, see Chapter 7.

HYPERTENSION (HIGH BLOOD PRESSURE)

Hypertension is a very serious health condition that is widely prevalent, under-recognized, and undertreated.

Blood pressure is measured in millimeters of mercury (mm Hg), and hypertension reflects pressure that is above the ideal.

What Should Your Blood Pressure Be?

A new set of blood-pressure guidelines for both health-care professionals and patients was issued by national experts in 2003 (the most recent year that guidelines were produced). They are as follows:

BLOOD-PRESSURE CLASSIFICATION	Systolic Blood Pressure (mm Hg)	Diastolic Blood Pressure (mm Hg)
Normal	<120	and <80
Pre-hypertension	120-139	or 80-89
Stage I Hypertension	140-159	or 90-99
Stage 2 Hypertension	≥160	or ≥100

http://www.nhlbi.nih.gov/guidelines/hypertension/express.pdf

The guidelines establish a normal blood pressure of 120/80 mm Hg. Some people with hypertension can attain this goal with regular exercise, an ideal body weight, and a meticulous diet. However, many people can't attain an ideal blood pressure even with these methods.

In these instances, medication can help. Often, more than one medication may be necessary to lower blood pressure satisfactorily.

There are numerous medications available to treat elevated blood pressure, and the most appropriate regimen is determined by collaboration between you and your physician. If you are prescribed a medication that you feel is causing side effects, let your physician know. There are other choices available.

Or if the medication seems too expensive, ask whether there is another equally good medicine that might cost less. Don't be discouraged if it requires two or even three medications to achieve your blood-pressure goals. The number of medications is not important. Instead, focus on the importance of attaining and maintaing a normal blood pressure!

There may be additional benefits to medication for high blood pressure if you have other heath problems. For instance, if you are diabetic, a group of medications called ACE inhibitors will help lower your blood pressure and also confer protection to your kidneys. If you have suffered a heart attack in the past, beta blockers are known to help reduce the risk of future heart attacks and sudden cardiac death. (See Chapter 7 for more on these medications.)

Hypertension also adversely affects organs besides the heart.

- *Aortic aneurysms* are seen with a greater frequency in hypertensive patients since the elevated pressures exert a heightened stress on the arterial vessel wall.

- *Strokes* are also more common.

- Hypertension can also disrupt the lining of the arterial wall, creating an environment for accelerated cholesterol deposits and blockages. The result is a heightened frequency of coronary artery atherosclerosis, leading to an increased risk of heart attacks. In fact, untreated hypertension is an important risk factor for *coronary artery disease.*

WHY TREAT HIGH BLOOD PRESSURE?

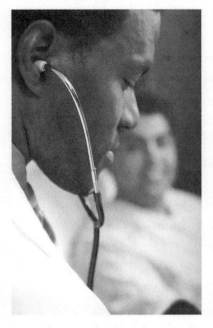

Why is lowering your blood pressure so important? After all, it doesn't cause any symptoms initially and furthermore doesn't interfere with your daily life.

Although this may be true, hypertension is called "the silent killer," and for good reason. Don't be fooled. A lack of symptoms doesn't mean that you are healthy. In fact, you are at great risk of future health problems.

Elevated blood pressure places an undue stress on the heart and the entire vascular system since the heart must pump against a heightened resistance to blood output. Over time, the heart will thicken.

Thickening heart muscle can predispose you to heart-rhythm disturbances and impair the ability of the heart to relax ("diastolic dysfunction"). As mentioned previously, abnormal relaxation of the heart can render higher pressures within the heart, further reducing its pumping efficiency.

If high blood pressure should go untreated for years, the heart muscle will begin to weaken and the heart chambers will enlarge ("systolic dysfunction," affecting the pumping of the heart). When systolic dysfunction is discovered, it is imperative that medication for high blood pressure be started immediately in order to:

- Prevent further deterioration of heart function
- Help reduce the workload on the weakened heart muscle
- Optimize the possibility of reversing heart-muscle dysfunction

● Hypertension also has a negative impact on *kidney function*. The heightened pressure directly damages the kidney tissue, rendering it less capable of filtering waste products from the bloodstream. Hypertension is the leading cause of kidney disease requiring dialysis.

Hypertension is completely preventable with proper blood-pressure screening and, when indicated, anti-hypertensive medication.

HYPERTROPHIC CARDIOMYOPATHY

Hypertrophic cardiomyopathy is a highly abnormal form of heart-muscle thickening that occurs independently of hypertension. Often, the left ventricle is severely thickened. The right ventricle may also be affected.

Heredity may play a part in some circumstances, so family members of an affected individual should be screened by echocardiography, an external ultrasound examination of the heart.

Patients with hypertrophic cardiomyopathy are subject to heart-rhythm disturbances and have an increased risk of sudden cardiac death. Patients may also suffer from syncope (fainting) and angina pectoris (chest pain).

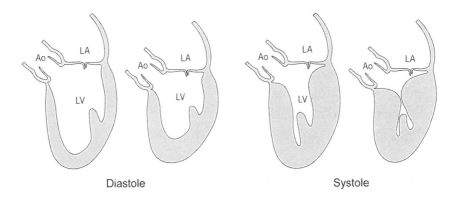

Diastole   Systole

In diastole, patients with hypertrophic cardiomyopathy demonstrate abnormal heart relaxation and elevated pressure within the heart. During systole, the opposing heart walls come in contact, impairing the output of blood from the heart. This can heighten heart pressure further, increasing lung congestion and symptoms of breathlessness.

Given the severe thickening of the left ventricle, the opposing walls may directly abut each other during the heart's contraction. This abutment causes a temporary interruption of systemic blood flow, including a reduction of blood flow to the brain and to the coronary arteries.

Furthermore, the advanced thickening of the left ventricle and the increased left ventricular pressure within the heart reduce effective coronary artery blood flow to the innermost left ventricular regions.

There are three effective methods to treat hypertrophic cardiomyopathy.

- Medications aimed at simultaneously reducing the force of the heart's contraction and slowing the heartbeat reduce the degree of left ventricular wall apposition.

- "Myectomy," an open-heart procedure in which a portion of the thickened left ventricle is surgically removed, is effective in advanced cases in which patients still have symptoms despite maximal drug therapy.

- A new procedure, alcohol ablation, is also surfacing at experienced medical centers. During this procedure, a carefully placed catheter is used to deliver a small amount of a sterile, alcohol-containing solution into a coronary artery that subserves the thickened region (the intraventricular septal region) of the left ventricle. This creates a purposeful limited heart attack, which causes regression or contraction of the thickness of the left ventricular wall and scarring of the heart muscle in this previously thickened region.

This chemically induced heart attack is very mild and does not negatively affect overall heart function. The patient is not at higher risk for a subsequent heart attack either. On the contrary, the objective of the procedure is to reduce the symptoms of hypertrophic cardiomyopathy, predominantly exertional shortness of breath and fatigue.

Usually, these methods reduce the previously impaired outflow of blood from the left ventricle, effectively diminishing and often eliminating symptoms that limit the patient's quality of life.

MITRAL INSUFFICIENCY

The mitral valve is one of four cardiac valves that direct blood flow within the heart, maintaining efficient oxygen transport to the body's vital organs and tissues. The mitral valve is positioned on the oxygen-rich left side of the heart, situated between the left upper chamber of the heart, the left atrium, and the left ventricle.

The mitral valve is composed of two thin leaflets, opening and closing approximately 100,000 times per day. Threadlike supporting structures called "chordae tendineae" assist with the normal opening and closing of the mitral valve leaflets.

The left atrium receives oxygen-rich blood from the four pulmonary veins. This blood is transmitted to the left ventricle during cardiac relaxation (a process known as "diastole") through an open mitral valve. During contraction of the left ventricle ("systole"), the mitral valve closes, with systemic blood flowing through an open aortic valve.

During cardiac systole, the mitral valve leaflets prolapse into the left atrium (see arrows, right), rendering the valve insufficient with a residual leaflet opening.

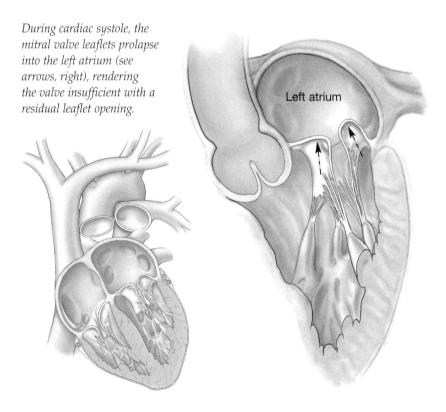

Left atrium

Under normal conditions, mitral valve blood flows in one direction. Therefore no blood flows from the left ventricle to the left atrium. With mitral insufficiency (known as "mitral regurgitation"), there is some ret- rograde (backward) blood flow from the left ventricle to the left atrium.

Ultrasound examinations of the heart can readily determine the quantity, direction, and mechanism of the mitral regurgitation. Small degrees of mitral insufficiency are frequently found at the time of echocardiography and are not generally problematic. Moderate to severe degrees of mitral insufficiency, however, require attention. An insufficient mitral valve results in the retrograde transport of blood from the high-pressure left ventricle to the low-pressure left atrium. This retrograde flow causes increased pressures within the left atrium and can result in a dilated left atrium. Over time, the increased pres- sures impede the delivery of oxygen-rich blood from the pulmonary veins to the left atrium, and increased lung pressures and CHF may develop as a result. The increased pressure within the left atrium and the dilatation of the left atrium also predispose the patient to such heart-rhythm abnormalities as atrial fibrillation and atrial flutter.

In advanced cases, the inefficient bidirectional blood flow across the mitral valve creates a volume overload of blood within the left ventricle. If severe and not corrected surgically, this overload can cause progressive left ventricular enlargement and dysfunction. This is a second mechanism for development of congestive heart failure.

There are several causes of mitral insufficiency.

- One well-known cause is mitral valve prolapse (described later in this chapter).

- Bacterial endocarditis, an infection on the mitral valve leaflets (described above), disrupts the structural integrity of the mitral valve leaflets.

- A cause of severe mitral insufficiency is a flail mitral valve leaflet, produced by a rupture of the chordae tendineae. This rupturing disrupts the structural integrity of the mitral valve and its ability to close, hence the term "flail" (unrestricted motion). The failure to close properly leaves a residual opening, causing a severe leakage.

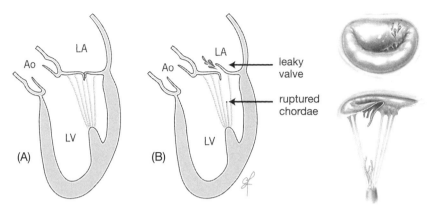

(A) Normal mitral valve closure
(B) A flail mitral leaflet produced by a rupture of the chordae tendineae

- Acute rheumatic fever, a streptococcus infection that occurs most often during childhood, may result in mitral insufficiency and mitral stenosis (see page 115) as aftereffects that appear decades later in adult life. (The immediate inflammatory response to acute rheumatic fever is called "valvulitis.")

The classic symptoms of advanced mitral insufficiency include shortness of breath, reduced exertional tolerance, palpitations, and cardiac irregularity that reflects underlying rhythm abnormalities such as frequent premature contractions, atrial flutter, and atrial fibrillation. In advanced and longstanding cases, fluid accumulation from congestive heart failure is present.

The most effective treatment of symptomatic mitral insufficiency is surgery to repair or replace the mitral valve. There are no medications known to be effective in reversing or attenuating advanced mitral insufficiency.

MITRAL VALVE PROLAPSE

Normally, the mitral valve closes during all of systole (ventricular contraction) with the two mitral valve leaflets forming a blood-tight seal that separates the left atrium from the left ventricle. During systole, when one or both mitral valve leaflets bow or "prolapse" into the left atrium, this event is termed "mitral valve prolapse."

Frequently, prolapsing of one or both mitral valve leaflets results in a lack of "coaptation," or coming together of the leaflets during ventricular systole. The prolapse results in some degree of mitral insufficiency, or valve leakage, creating a bidirectional pattern of blood flow across the mitral valve. As a consequence, an inefficient state of blood flow – back and forth instead of in one direction – is created.

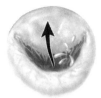

Leaky closure

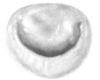

Normal closure

With mitral valve prolapse, the valve leaflets are often thickened and floppy (also known as "redundant"). The cause is not certain but may be related to abnormality in tissues that connect to and compose the valve leaflets. The mitral insufficiency creates turbulent and high-velocity blood flow into the left atrium. With a stethoscope, the physician hears this turbulent blood flow over the chest wall as a heart murmur.

In extreme situations, mitral valve prolapse can result in severe mitral insufficiency. (See page 115.) If mitral valve prolapse has been present for a long time, or if the mitral valve apparatus weakens and becomes disrupted (causing sudden severe mitral insufficiency), as with a ruptured

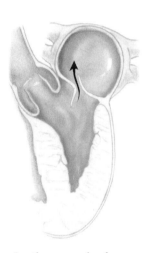

Another example of a flail mitral valve leaflet with mitral valve regurgitation (arrows)

chordae, precipitous congestive heart failure with accumulation of fluid within the lungs may ensue. Fortunately, this latter scenario is not common.

Not all prolapsing valves leak to a significant degree. But as noted above, one or more chordae may rupture, possibly from the stress of being stretched for many years by the prolapsed valve. When these chordae rupture, insufficiency can progress from mild to severe fairly quickly, as the valve may become flail.

There are no known effective medications to reverse advanced mitral insufficiency. Mitral valve prolapse that causes symptoms, together with moderately severe to severe mitral insufficiency, must be treated by surgery.

Unlike other causes of mitral insufficiency, prolapsing mitral valves can most often be repaired, thus avoiding the need to replace the valve.

Surgery is done in the traditional open-heart manner. The postoperative hospital stay is usually five days, and under most circumstances full recovery can be expected within six to eight weeks.

The risks associated with mitral valve repair are the same as those connected with any open-heart surgery – stroke, heart attack, death, infection, heart-rhythm disturbances, and pleural effusion (fluid collection on the lungs). Fortunately, these occurrences are quite rare and the benefits clearly outweigh the risks in properly selected patients. In fact, in experienced health-care centers, the mortality (death) rates are far less than a few percent, often approaching zero.

Following the surgery, it's important to keep track of how you're feeling and the activities you're able to perform. Be sure you know the answers to the following questions when you are going to see your cardiologist.

- Is your incision healing? Or is it red and inflamed?
- Is there any discharge from the incision?
- Can you exercise?
- Is your strength improving?
- Are your walking distance and time improving, or do you have shortness of breath?
- Do you perceive an abnormal heart rhythm?
- Do you have ankle swelling to indicate that you are retaining fluid?
- Is your breathing worse, especially when you're lying down?
- Are you experiencing precipitous weight gain that diet alone can't explain (but which would suggest fluid accumulation)?
- How's your blood pressure?
- Do you have fevers or chills?

Call your cardiologist if your answer is yes to any of these questions; it may indicate that you're regressing after surgery. Keep in mind that most people recover extremely satisfactorily.

MYOCARDIAL INFARCTION (HEART ATTACK)

A myocardial infarction (MI, or heart attack) is caused by inadequate blood flow to the heart's left ventricle. In most myocardial infarctions, a buildup of coronary atherosclerotic plaque becomes unstable and fissures. A thrombus, which is a combination of blood products (blood clot), abruptly forms on the fissured plaque, creating an abrupt obstruction of the artery. This obstruction blocks blood flow to a region of the heart's left ventricle. This abrupt disruption of regional blood flow to the heart often results in heart-muscle cell death and irreversible damage to the left ventricle, as seen on an echocardiogram.

A myocardial infarction can also occur without a completely blocked artery. Temperature extremes, high levels of exertion, illnesses such as high fevers, or recent noncardiac surgery may increase the heart's need for oxygen. This increased demand, however, may outstrip the diminished supply if you have an advanced but incomplete blockage. Under these circumstances, the imbalance of oxygen supply and demand can result in a myocardial infarction. Furthermore, the coronary arteries may spasm to cause a myocardial infarction. Spasm may occur when a person uses illicit substances such as cocaine.

The symptoms of a heart attack are central or left-sided chest pressure, discomfort, or pain. The discomfort often radiates to other locations, including the throat, neck, jaw, teeth, and the inner aspect of the left and right arms. These symptoms reflect insufficient oxygen delivery to the heart's left ventricle. Other symptoms may include shortness of breath, a sense of doom, sweating, nausea, and both fast and slow heart rates.

Treatment: Time Is Heart Muscle

Treatment of a myocardial infarction attempts to restore blood flow to the heart as soon as possible. Time is essential, as regaining normal blood flow will limit the amount of damage that the heart incurs. Two treatment methods are used to restore blood flow in a timely manner.

- ### THROMBOLYTIC MEDICATIONS ("CLOT-BUSTERS")

One modality is to administer an IV medication called a "thrombolytic." Thrombolytic IV medications "lyse" or break up the coronary blood clot a high percentage of the time. Blood-thinning IV medications are frequently administered at the same time as the thrombolytic. Neither the thrombolytic medication nor the adjunctive blood-thinning agents affects the underlying atherosclerotic plaque.

Hemorrhagic bleeding in the brain and bleeding elsewhere is a slight risk of thrombolytic therapy.

After thrombolytic therapy, expect to spend two to three days in the hospital for observation, as you would for a heart attack. To monitor whether the thrombolytic medications have opened up the artery, you will probably have a series of ECGs. Your blood will be drawn and your cardiac enzymes measured.

If the thrombolytics were effective at opening the artery, you'll have a rapid rise and a higher peak of your cardiac enzymes because of the "washout phenomenon," which means that the injured muscle is washed out with the restoration of blood flow. The enzymes will enter the bloodstream more quickly and therefore their levels will peak earlier. Follow-up is basically the same as after a heart attack. (See page 124.)

- ### ANGIOPLASTY AND STENT

The second effective modality to restore blood flow immediately includes percutaneous transluminal coronary angioplasty (PTCA) and stent placement.

Briefly, PTCA uses a tiny inflatable balloon attached to a catheter. The deflated balloon is placed across the atherosclerotic plaque and inflated, increasing the size of the lumen (the channel through the artery), thereby improving blood flow.

A stent, a small wire mesh-like device, is also introduced by a similar catheter technique and permanently deployed (placed) within the arterial segment where the atherosclerotic obstruction was previously cleared by PTCA.

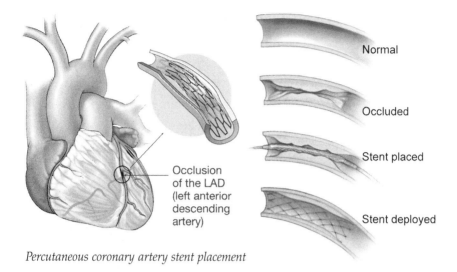

Normal

Occluded

Stent placed

Stent deployed

Occlusion
of the LAD
(left anterior
descending
artery)

Percutaneous coronary artery stent placement

The stents buttress the coronary artery, pushing and compressing the atherosclerotic plaque against the vessel wall.

PTCA and stent placement are useful techniques for stabilizing a patient during a myocardial infarction and mitigating further damage to the left ventricle. When there are a number of severe coronary artery obstructions, a future coronary artery bypass grafting surgery may still be needed.

The importance of staying on an antiplatelet medicine such as clopidogrel after stent placement cannot be overstated, especially if you have received a "drug-eluting" stent (a stent that releases a pharmacological agent to prevent reblockage). Current guidelines recommend a minimum of one year of clopidogrel following a stent procedure with a drug-eluting stent, and some physicians believe that three or four years, or even a lifetime of clopidogrel, will be necessary to avoid a complication called "stent thrombosis."

In stent thrombosis, clots can form within the stent because the artery's lining (endothelium) may not have healed completely, resulting in inability to ward off such thrombus formation.

If you have a bare metal stent implanted instead of a drug-eluting one, then a minimum of three months of clopidogrel is recommended. (These recommendations are evolving as more data emerge on the risks of stent thrombosis.)

If you need to have an unrelated surgery, for example gall-bladder surgery following the stent placement, you may need to stop your clopidogrel temporarily (to reduce your risk of bleeding from the surgery). However, stopping temporarily can increase your risk of stent thrombosis.

If you do have surgery scheduled, you must call your cardiologist first so a plan to stop your clopidogrel can be developed. Unless you face a surgical emergency, your surgeon or the anesthesiologist should NOT stop the medication without consulting your cardiologist. While you're off the clopidogrel, you may need "bridging" with another form of blood-thinner, such as heparin.

This bridging may even require a brief hospitalization. It is not known for certain that bridging with heparin therapy will entirely mitigate the risk of temporarily stopping clopidogrel.

CORONARY ARTERY BYPASS GRAFTING (CABG)

If necessary, CABG can be performed on an emergency basis. This would require a heart catheterization to determine the location of the coronary artery blockages.

A CABG operation would most often be recommended in an emergency setting if several life-threatening blockages were discovered and were deemed too high risk or not amenable to angioplasty or stenting. Fortunately, this is not a common scenario.

Cardiogenic Shock

Significant sudden damage to the heart muscle may create a medical emergency called "cardiogenic shock." In cases of extensive damage, the weakened heart muscle cannot generate sufficient blood flow to the peripheral tissues and organs. When cardiogenic shock happens, emergent opening of the blocked coronary artery with PTCA (see page 121, percutaneous transluminal coronary angioplasty), with or without stent placement, offers the best chance for survival.

The severe nature of cardiogenic shock requires closer and more frequent post-hospitalization follow-up, possibly including a number of medications that need to be adjusted periodically. This is because you'll be at a higher risk to develop congestive heart failure, significant heart dysfunction, and heart-rhythm disturbances. If after several months of such aggressive care your heart function does not improve sufficiently, you would become a candidate for a defibrillator to lessen the risk of sudden cardiac death.

POST-HEART-ATTACK CARE

A number of preventive measures are undertaken after a heart attack. Perhaps the most important is stopping use of all tobacco products. Normalizing blood pressure is extremely important. A persistently elevated blood pressure exerts extra work on an already damaged heart.

Normalizing blood pressure is typically achieved through a combination of diet and weight loss; a regular, initially supervised program of exercise; and carefully selected prescription medications. Achieving normal blood lipids with appropriate ratios of total cholesterol, HDL cholesterol, and LDL cholesterol also remains a priority.

Medications will be prescribed to help you achieve your lipid goals and to prevent or delay further heart damage after a myocardial infarction. (Lipid medications are discussed in Chapter 7.)

- *HMG Co-A reductase inhibitors,* called "statins," partially block the production of cholesterol in the liver, principally reducing total cholesterol and LDL cholesterol blood levels. Through an alternative mechanism, perhaps an anti-inflammatory effect at the site of the coronary artery plaque, these agents help to stabilize plaque, preventing it from rupturing and causing another heart attack. (Vascular inflammation appears to play an integral role in promoting both the formation of atherosclerotic plaque and its instability, making it prone to rupture and cause heart attacks. Further understanding of this process will most likely assist in preventing heart attacks.) Through carefully controlled research studies, statins have been shown to reduce the risks of repeat myocardial infarctions and death.

- *Aspirin* serves as an antiplatelet agent. Since platelets are the main blood-clotting component of blood, to render platelets inactive results in blood-thinning. The blood-thinning action is believed to reduce the incidence of abrupt thrombus formation at the site of a cholesterol plaque within the coronary artery.

- *Beta blockers* block the effects of adrenaline at the tissue level. They reduce heart rate and blood pressure, resulting in less work for the heart, reduced oxygen requirements, and reduced oxygen consumption, all beneficial in patients who have obstructions in their coronary arteries and who have suffered a heart attack.

- *ACE inhibitors* have been found in recent studies to reduce the incidence of a repeat heart attack and death in patients who have already had a heart attack. They also reduce the incidence of heart-aneurysm formation.

Following your heart attack, be aware of any new signs and symptoms that may develop, monitor your capacity to exert yourself, and record your weight daily. If your physical capacity has plateaued at a suboptimal level or is regressing, alert your cardiologist.

Rapid weight gain may indicate fluid retention. Other symptoms to watch for include pulse rates that are irregular or inappropriate to the activity in which you're engaging, lightheadedness, or fainting or near-fainting. Be sure to call your cardiologist when such symptoms occur.

PALPITATIONS

Palpitations are a subjective feeling of heart-fluttering, rapid heartbeats, and/or early heartbeats. Most commonly, palpitations signal early or premature heartbeats originating from either the atria or ventricles. Premature heartbeats originating from the atria are termed "premature atrial complexes" (PACs) and those originating from the ventricles are termed "premature ventricular complexes" (PVCs).

Palpitations may or may not be a sign of heart disease. Both PACs and PVCs are common under normal circumstances and occur more often in persons who drink alcohol or caffeine excessively. Other precipitating factors include physical or emotional stress and poor sleep habits.

Premature heartbeats may also arise from underlying structural heart disease. Heart-muscle thickening and an enlargement of cardiac chambers are often the consequence of blood pressure that has remained high for an extended time. These changes render the patient more susceptible to heart-rhythm disturbances, including premature heartbeats. Similar to high blood pressure, valvular heart disease and a previous heart attack can have an adverse impact on the heart's structure, creating the substrate for heart arrhythmias.

PACs and PVCs may be harbingers of serious heart-rhythm disturbances, such as atrial fibrillation, atrial flutter, and ventricular tachycardia (see page 135), particularly in the setting of structural heart disease. For this reason, any new symptoms of heart arrhythmia may merit a cardiac evaluation to assess for structural heart disease (electrocardiogram and echocardiogram) and coronary artery disease (stress-testing).

If these tests are abnormal, especially if the stress test suggests the possibility of underlying coronary blockage, it is likely that you will be referred for cardiac catheterization.

PERICARDITIS

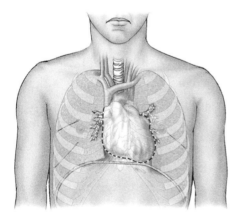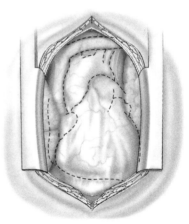

The pericardium is a thin lining covering the heart. Within the pericardial sac, a small amount of fluid is present to reduce the friction over the heart surface during its contraction and movement.

The pericardium is a thin-walled sac that surrounds the heart and great vessels in the central chest cavity, termed the "mediastinum." The pericardium normally contains approximately one ounce (25-50 milliliters) of fluid. The purpose of this fluid is to reduce the friction between the contracting heart and the mediastinal structures. The pericardium is actually two layers. The first layer is composed of the sac and the second layer is attached to the external heart surface. These layers are respectively called the parietal and visceral pericardium.

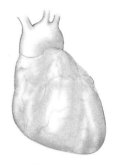

Normal

When diseased, the pericardium may become inflamed. Inflammation of the pericardium creates friction between the two pericardial layers, interfering with its lubricating function. It can restrict normal heart motion, and its inflamed layers can lose their ability to dispense with the normal pericardial fluid, at times culminating in large collections of fluid. An excess of pericardial

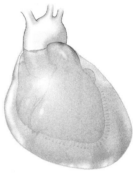

Effusion

Pericardial effusion – an excess of pericardial fluid

fluid is termed a "pericardial effusion." Large collections of pericardial fluid can compress the heart's structures, impairing the filling of the cardiac chambers with blood and severely reducing outflow of blood from the heart. A large pericardial effusion can be a medical emergency requiring prompt elimination of the collected pericardial fluid either by a small needle inserted through the skin under local anesthesia or a small surgical incision under deeper anesthesia.

Symptoms of pericarditis include chest pain, typically sharp pain that worsens when you inhale or lie flat. The pain may travel to the back, particularly at the shoulder blade level. It can be confused with a heart attack. The pain can be partly relieved by leaning forward, which may lessen the contact between the two layers of inflamed pericardial tissue. Tests for pericarditis include an electrocardiogram, which can demonstrate electrical signs of pericardial inflammation, and echocardiography to look for evidence of a thickened pericardium and an abnormal accumulation of pericardial fluid.

Fortunately, pericarditis is uncommon. The most common cause is open-heart surgery, when we open the pericardium to gain access to heart structures. The most common nonsurgical cause of pericardial inflammation is viral pericarditis. For uncertain reasons, a common virus that causes an upper respiratory infection or cold can infrequently inflame the pericardium. Less common causes are a bacterial infection, malignancy, or systemic arthritis such as rheumatoid arthritis.

The mainstay of pericarditis treatment is anti-inflammatory medication such as ibuprofen. Appropriate antibiotics are prescribed when a bacterial infection is confirmed. Pain medication is often necessary and recovery is generally routine. Recurrences can occur but do so rarely.

PERIPHERAL VASCULAR DISEASE

Peripheral vascular disease is a manifestation of the same atherosclerotic process found in the coronary arteries. The only difference is the location. All atherosclerotic arterial disease outside the heart is termed peripheral vascular disease.

- The carotid arteries – the main arteries in the neck that serve as large conduits for oxygenated blood flow to the brain – are commonly affected.
- Another territory commonly involved is the aorta, the main blood vessel leaving the heart and delivering oxygen-rich blood to the remainder of the body.
- Beyond the aorta, arteries in the legs are also frequently involved with atherosclerosis.

The numerous vascular territories subject to atherosclerosis highlight an important fact. Atherosclerosis is a systemic or "total body" process. Once atherosclerosis is identified in one vascular territory, it means that atherosclerosis is present to some extent throughout the entire vascular system.

If significant atherosclerosis is detected in your carotid arteries, for example, it is important that you be screened for significant atherosclerosis involving other organ systems, such as the heart, legs, and the abdominal aorta.

Screening the abdominal aorta can consist of palpating (feeling) the aorta for enlargement or performing an abdominal ultrasound, which is a painless, noninvasive, risk-free test. With the heart, stress-testing may be important. If atherosclerosis is suspected in the legs, your doctor will check your leg pulses during a physical examination and measure the blood pressure in each leg to calculate your ankle-brachial index (a measure of the fall of blood pressure in the arteries supplying the legs).

Symptoms connected with your legs, such as your calves burning (claudication) with exercise, profound leg fatigue with less than maximal levels of activity, or open wounds or nonhealing ulcers on your feet are all cause for concern, as they suggest peripheral vascular disease and reduced oxygen delivery to vital tissues in the feet and legs.

Treatment

Treatment for peripheral vascular disease begins with reduction of risk factors. This means:

- Quitting smoking
- Control of blood lipids
- Blood pressure control
- A healthy diet
- Increased activity

Exercise can actually improve blood flow to the legs by helping to recruit the formation of what are called collateral vessels, new blood vessels that form to bypass the obstruction and bring more blood to the legs.

Cilostazol is a medication used to treat the symptoms of peripheral vascular disease, but it can't be taken if you have CHF.

Other options include angioplasty/stenting and bypass operations of the lower extremities, similar to those that are performed for patients with coronary artery blockages.

If you have peripheral vascular disease, you should monitor the progression of your symptoms as well as leg and foot wounds that aren't healing. Oxygen is required for wounds to heal, and if you have peripheral vascular disease, the oxygen supply to your extremities is compromised. Unhealed wounds can threaten toes or limbs if not addressed.

It's extremely important that you wear socks and shoes, even in the house, to decrease the risk of foot wounds. You will also need to maintain meticulous preventive care, which includes seeing a podiatrist regularly for proper foot and toenail care.

PREMATURE ATRIAL CONTRACTION

A premature atrial contraction (PAC) is a premature heartbeat. In PACs, the heart's electrical impulse originates in either the left or right atrium (upper chambers) outside the region of the normal pacemaker, the sinus node.

By definition, a PAC is premature, occurring before the next sinus-node discharge. This premature electrical impulse then travels to the heart's lower chambers, resulting in the premature or early contraction of both the right and left ventricles.

Since this contraction is early, the heart has not had its normal amount of time to fill with blood. Therefore the heart's output of blood immediately following a PAC is less, resulting in the transmission of a weaker pulse, easily felt at the wrist as both earlier and less forceful than normal.

There are numerous causes of PACs:

- Overactive thyroid gland
- Anemia
- Infection
- Sleep deprivation
- Alcohol use
- Caffeine ingestion
- Nicotine use
- Increased emotion

PACs may precede other cardiac rhythm abnormalities such as atrial fibrillation.

Single PACs are not dangerous. Three or more PACs in rapid succession are classified as paroxysmal atrial tachycardia. This is not particularly dangerous because each occurrence of the heart-rhythm disturbance typically lasts a few seconds at most.

Prolonged and consecutive PACs may cause the heart to contract less efficiently, reducing the output of blood from the heart. This reduction in output may result in symptoms of lightheadedness, although rarely.

Prolonged and consecutive PACs may cause the heart to contract less efficiently, reducing the output of blood from the heart.

Most often, PACs are viewed as merely a nuisance. The most frequent symptom is a perceived heart flutter or thumping that lasts a few seconds. Heart flutter may be annoying and affect your ability to concentrate.

Often, PACs are noticed soon after you go to bed, following an abrupt change in position coupled with a sudden lack of external stimulation as your ear is pressed against your pillow. When this happens, awareness of your heartbeat pattern is greater because the heartbeat is transmitted to your ear with increased ease.

First-line treatment of PACs is lifestyle modification. Use of nicotine and alcohol should be reduced – preferably eliminated – and regular sleep patterns should be established. Should symptomatic PACs persist despite improvements to your lifestyle, your physician may prescribe a beta blocker. Beta blockers blunt the cardiac effects of circulating adrenaline, reducing the electrical irritability of the heart rhythm.

If you're feeling better on the beta blocker and the PACs are less frequent once you're on the medicine, follow-up is infrequent – perhaps yearly – to ensure that your ECG has not changed and that you're still able to tolerate the beta blocker.

PACs that are the result of an illness are generally temporary and tend to cease once the illness has resolved.

PREMATURE VENTRICULAR CONTRACTIONS

Premature ventricular contractions, or PVCs, are similar to PACs except that the premature electrical depolarization originates in either of the two lower cardiac chambers, the left or right ventricle. As with PACs, PVCs are more of a nuisance provided that you don't have damage to the heart's structure.

Frequent PVCs in the setting of reduced heart function, such as in patients with a previous heart attack or a viral cardiomyopathy, may portend a more serious heart-rhythm disturbance such as ventricular tachycardia. (See page 135.) This requires careful consultation with your physician, who may recommend an electrophysiology study and/or implantable cardiac defibrillator placement.

RHEUMATIC HEART DISEASE

Rheumatic fever is a result of a throat infection caused by the group A streptococcus bacteria, an illness that most often affects children. Rheumatic fever affects the heart as well as other parts of the body, often scarring the valves so that the heart has to work harder to pump blood.

Over decades, the valves progressively degenerate, resulting in both a restricted opening of the valve leaflets (stenosis) and incomplete closure, which results in valve leakage (regurgitation).

If you have only mild or moderate manifestations of rheumatic heart disease, you'll be followed yearly with an echocardiogram and a physical examination.

If you have more advanced or severe rheumatic heart disease, you should be seen every six months for a physical exam, symptomatic reassessment, and an echocardiogram.

Your heart rhythm will also be followed closely with a series of electrocardiograms. Patients with rheumatic heart disease are prone to develop heart-rhythm disturbances, particularly atrial rhythm disturbances (most commonly atrial fibrillation/flutter).

If you develop significant symptoms, such as difficulty exerting yourself, shortness of breath, swelling of the lower extremities, or signs of elevated pressure in the lungs (pulmonary hypertension), you will be considered for valve repair or more likely valve-replacement surgery, because repair may be difficult when the valves are severely degenerated, inflamed, and scarred.

SUDDEN CARDIAC DEATH

Sudden cardiac death is a tragic manifestation of heart disease. As the term suggests, death is sudden and unexpected, with a cardiac cause.

The most common cause of sudden cardiac death is a heart-rhythm disturbance secondary to obstructive coronary artery disease. When a total coronary artery blockage occurs suddenly, oxygen delivery to the heart stops abruptly. This cessation of oxygen delivery can result in dangerous heart-rhythm disturbances such as ventricular tachycardia and ventricular fibrillation. Because of these disturbances, the output of blood is not sufficient to provide adequate oxygen delivery to the brain, producing unconsciousness and death if cardiopulmonary resuscitation (CPR) is not attempted or is unsuccessful.

Sudden cardiac death also results from chronic coronary artery disease. In persons who have suffered a previous heart attack, the border zone between normal and scarred heart tissue is "arrhythmogenic," meaning that it can foster the genesis of a heart-rhythm disturbance.

This is especially true of more severe heart attacks, in which residual heart function is at least moderately impaired. Patients with significant heart-muscle weakening from a previous heart attack are at the highest risk of sudden death, and often merit preemptive placement of an implantable cardiac defibrillator.

Other causes of sudden cardiac death include advanced valvular heart disease and certain toxins, including illicit drugs.

Sudden cardiac death is preventable in many cases. To reduce its likelihood, aggressive efforts are presently underway to identify high-risk patients, ensuring that they be placed on the best medications coupled with placement of an implantable cardiac defibrillator (ICD).

An ICD is a small electronic device that can be put into your chest without open-heart surgery. It monitors the heart rhythm.

When a life-threatening abnormal rhythm occurs – most commonly ventricular tachycardia (see page 135) – the ICD will "recognize" it and start pacing the heart at a higher rate than that of the ventricular tachycardia itself. This "overdrive" function of the pacemaker portion of the ICD suppresses and often eradicates the abnormal rhythm.

If the overdrive pacing is not successful in converting the arrhythmia to a normal heart rhythm after a preprogrammed period of time, then the defibrillator will "know" to deliver an internal shock to restore a normal rhythm.

The ICD is periodically checked for such rhythm disturbances, especially ventricular arrhythmias, since it has a memory capability. The number of such episodes that are terminated by the device is also recorded. These checks can be made over your telephone line every few months.

You will need to be seen every 6 to 12 months at a minimum for a more complete in-person defibrillator evaluation.

SYNCOPE

Syncope refers to the loss of consciousness. It results from a reduction of blood flow to the brain. Syncope can be a minor event, for example as a transient reaction to having your blood drawn. It can also be quite serious, due to an abnormal heart-rhythm disturbance during an acute heart attack, causing sudden cardiac death.

Syncope may be postural, related to standing for a long time. In fact, most cases can be explained by prolonged standing and/or dehydration.

Most occurrences can be minimized or avoided by:

- Adequate fluid intake
- Avoiding standing in one spot for prolonged periods
- Increasing dietary sodium intake
- Wearing compression stockings

The cardiac causes of syncope (such as serious heart-rhythm disturbances) are the ones that merit careful evaluation and treatment to prevent both an occurrence and recurrence. (See "Sudden Cardiac Death," page 133.)

VENTRICULAR TACHYCARDIA

Ventricular tachycardia is an abnormally fast cardiac rhythm originating in either the left or right lower chamber (ventricle) of the heart. This abnormal heart rhythm most often occurs from a single location in the ventricle, in which an irritable electrical focus (the precise site within the heart's electrical system from which the arrhythmia originates) usurps the heart's normal rhythm.

Ventricular tachycardia is more serious than heart rhythms originating from the upper chambers of the heart, as heart rates may become extremely fast (greater than 200 beats per minute).

The fast heart rates coupled with the rhythm's location (left or right ventricle) may cause a significant impairment in blood output from the heart, dangerously low blood pressure, and reduced blood flow to the brain. Symptoms may include lightheadedness and fainting. Sudden death is a possibility if the arrhythmia persists and skilled CPR personnel are not present.

Ventricular tachycardia may be stable or unstable.

- In the stable form, you may be aware of a fast heart rate and may experience slight lightheadedness. There is no precipitous drop in blood pressure.
- The unstable form produces a significant drop in blood pressure and is usually considered a medical emergency.

The treatment of the stable form of ventricular tachycardia starts with IV antiarrhythmic medications aimed at converting the heart rhythm to normal. Should the IV medications not be successful, a direct current cardioversion (DCC) can be done. This treatment is highly successful at restoring the heart rhythm to normal. (See "Atrial Fibrillation," page 90, for a detailed description of DCC.)

In the unstable form of ventricular tachycardia, the patient is often unconscious and an electrical cardioversion is attempted on an emergency basis. The success rate of the electrical cardioversion in the unstable form of ventricular tachycardia is in part related to the length of time the heart has been in the abnormal rhythm. The longer the duration of the abnormal rhythm, the longer the heart has experienced reduced blood supply.

Closely coupled with the success of the cardioversion is the underlying condition of the heart muscle. If the heart muscle is severely weakened, perhaps from a previous major heart attack, the chances of successfully restoring the normal rhythm are significantly lower.

There are a number of causes of ventricular tachycardia. Most often, it is caused by coronary artery blockages. Previous heart attacks are common in many patients with coronary artery disease. The heart attack forms a scar within the heart. This scar serves as an irritable electrical focus, and it lowers the threshold for both inducing and sustaining ventricular tachycardia.

Even without a previous heart attack, coronary artery disease can lower the threshold for the occurrence of arrhythmias. Transient interruptions or imbalances of the oxygen supply to the heart, for instance, when oxygen supply is outstripped by demand, can generate electrical irritability and induce arrhythmias.

The following conditions also increase the risk of ventricular tachycardia:

- Valvular heart disease and heart-muscle weakening
- Hypertensive heart disease with a thickened heart muscle
- Heart-muscle weakening caused by a virus

In addition to treating ventricular tachycardia, it is important to prevent its recurrence. Since coronary artery disease is the most common cause, medications are prescribed to restore the balance between the heart muscle's supply of and demand for oxygen.

Beta blockers are the principal medications used for this purpose. They help achieve this desirable balance by blunting the heart rate with exertion. They also directly suppress the vigor with which the heart contracts. Both outcomes result from blocking the effects of circulating adrenaline.

Medications that lower blood pressure may also help. Reducing the blood pressure reduces the amount of oxygen that the heart requires to function.

Nitrates are another possibility. Oral nitrates are a long-acting form of nitroglycerin. Their main effect is to directly dilate the coronary arteries, thereby improving coronary artery blood flow when blockages are present. This effect is somewhat limited when the blockages are significant, because the blockages are relatively fixed and won't respond to the dilating properties of nitroglycerin.

Heart-rhythm medications may also be prescribed. Most often, these medications are started in the hospital with careful and continuous monitoring of the heart rhythm over the first 48 to 72 hours. This monitoring is necessary because paradoxically, some of these medications may actually precipitate an abnormal heart rhythm (termed a "pro-arrhythmia").

WOLFE-PARKINSON-WHITE SYNDROME

Wolfe-Parkinson-White syndrome is a congenital abnormality of the heart's electrical system. With Wolfe-Parkinson-White syndrome, there are one or more extra electrical connections between the upper and lower cardiac chambers. When an electrical impulse successfully traverses one or more of these "accessory pathways," it permits extremely fast conduction velocities, occasionally even up to 300 beats per minute.

In this situation, especially in a patient who also has atrial arrhythmias such as atrial flutter and atrial fibrillation, the heart rhythm can degenerate into ventricular fibrillation. Sudden death can ensue if efforts are not made to resuscitate the patient using CPR and/or a defibrillator.

This condition is most often found on a routine electrocardiogram. Patients successfully resuscitated from an episode of near sudden death may also be identified by electrocardiogram testing as having Wolfe-Parkinson-White syndrome.

The best and most definitive treatment is radiofrequency ablation of the accessory pathway, in which a catheter is placed in the bloodstream and is precisely guided to the accessory pathway location using electrical recordings within the heart. Subsequently, a small amount of radiofrequency energy is delivered, "burning" the pathway and disrupting its electrical conducting properties. (Radiofrequency ablation is discussed on page 92 in the section on atrial fibrillation.)

Medications can also be used but, unlike radiofrequency ablation, do not provide an effective cure. Instead, medications slow the conduction properties of the accessory pathway and reduce the frequency of the arrhythmia episodes.

If RFA has not been recommended to you, consider asking your doctor about it. ◆

Chapter 7

Understanding Your Cardiac Medications

Cardiac medications take many forms. It's vitally important to know what medications you are taking and the rationale for each.

It's part of my job to take the time and effort to fully explain my prescribing rationale to each patient in a clear, medically accurate manner. The patient then understands better why the medication is necessary, and the physician-patient relationship has been enhanced.

If we need to adjust the medication in the future, the patient will generally accept and endorse the changes more readily because of the previous explanation.

RISK VS. BENEFIT

I'd like to mention a common theme each physician and patient faces concerning health care in general and medication in particular: risk versus benefit. Does the benefit of the medication, by reducing morbidity (e.g., heart attack and stroke) and mortality (death rates) and simultaneously improving a patient's quality of life, outweigh the risks of side effects and the rare occurrence of an allergic reaction? Certainly the physician thinks the benefit is greater than the risk, or she wouldn't have written the prescription.

Sometimes a patient is hesitant to start taking a particular medication. Maybe a friend took it and had a negative reaction, or the patient read a list of potentially unpleasant side effects on the Internet.

I recommend that you discuss any such concerns with your doctor. The discussion can help you understand the rationale for the prescribed medication, its desired benefits, and the advantages to your health. Even if your doctor has already talked with you about the medication, don't hesitate to bring up any questions.

Some patients don't require lengthy explanations about the risks and benefits of medications and allergies. Instead, they arrive at the physician's office, ask for medical advice, endorse the opinion of the physician, and readily accept a prescription. After a brief explanation outlining the prescription rationale, they take the medication faithfully without performing independent research.

Other patients ask numerous questions, focus on extreme detail, and continue to perform their own research after leaving the office. These are the patients with whom I often assume proactive involvement, outlining in detail the indication for the prescription, the possible side effects, and their expected frequency.

A PICTURE IS WORTH
A THOUSAND WORDS

Either way, I find drawing simple and clear pictures extremely helpful. For instance, for a patient with a regurgitant or leaking mitral valve, I can best explain the prescription rationale for an angiotensin converting enzyme (ACE) inhibitor medication with a simple drawing of the heart.

An ACE inhibitor will dilate the peripheral arteries and reduce blood pressure. It can reduce the degree of mitral valve leakage. Also, it may delay and possibly prevent cardiac enlargement, heart-muscle weakening, and the need for reparative mitral valve surgery.

> With an explanation and drawing, even the most "medication-hesitant" patient is almost always willing to take medication as recommended.

With an explanation and drawing, even the most "medication-hesitant" patient is almost always willing to take medication as recommended.

BETA BLOCKERS

Beta receptors are located on cells in the heart and walls of the blood vessels. They normally serve as an attachment point for circulating adrenaline.

Circulating adrenaline raises the heart rate by directly stimulating the heart-muscle cells by binding to the beta receptors. Adrenaline also causes vascular muscle cells to contract, resulting in a narrowing of the arteries and an increase in blood pressure.

These actions are counterproductive in patients with heart disease. Raising the pulse rate and blood pressure increases the heart's work-load and therefore increases the stress on the heart. This added stress can be deleterious to heart function when oxygen delivery to the heart is reduced, as when coronary artery blockages are present.

Beta blockers block these receptors and in doing so they block the effects of circulating adrenaline. This reduces the vigor of heart contractility.

Beta blockers lower the resting pulse rate, and more important, they reduce the heart rate at a given level of exertion (similar to a miles-per-hour limiter on your car).

These combined actions reduce the work of the heart and its oxygen requirements. They are especially valuable if there is a structural defect in the heart, such as coronary artery disease.

Because of their anti-adrenaline effects, beta blockers can also favorably influence the heart rhythm. They reduce the likelihood of atrial and ventricular arrhythmias in patients who may be predisposed, such as those patients who have experienced a previous heart attack.

They also reduce blood pressure by enlarging (dilating) peripheral vessels, again a beneficial effect in most cardiac patients. If you have had a heart attack, beta blockers are an essential component of your pharmaceutical regimen, since they have been conclusively found to reduce the likelihood of future heart attack and sudden cardiac death. They reduce the risk of death by reducing the incidence of fatal heart-rhythm disturbances.

TODAY'S INTERNET: THE
MISINFORMATION HIGHWAY?

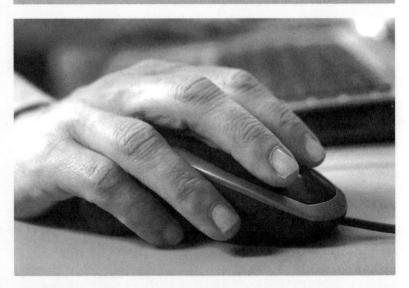

Given today's easy access to medical information, including medical books and data provided by doctors, pharmacists, and the Internet, many patients educate themselves about their medications.

Based on the information they find, patients sometimes are cautious about beginning newly prescribed medications. Understandably, the published lists of adverse reactions frightens them. I frequently have to remind my patients that many of the listed reactions are quite rare.

If you have any qualms about taking a medication as directed, talk openly with your doctor. You are entitled to a full explanation of the rationale for treatment, the expected benefits and possible risks of the medication, and the frequency of the risks occurring in research studies.

As I mentioned in Chapter 4, it's important to use highly reliable sites when you are doing medical research. In addition to the previously mentioned Cleveland Clinic and American Heart Association sites, you will find good content at:

- http://www.theheart.org/index.do
- http://www.womenheart.org
- http://www.webMD.com
- http://www.cdc.gov/heartdisease

Beta blockers are generally well tolerated, especially when initiated at modest doses that are increased gradually. The following side effects, however, have been observed with beta blockers.

- Fatigue
- Sexual dysfunction in men
- A worsening or exacerbation of asthma symptoms. Therefore, cautious starting doses are recommended in those with asthma.
- A masking of the symptoms of low blood sugar. In diabetic patients with a tendency toward unpredictably low blood sugars, beta blockers can be taken, but with caution. Consult your physician.
- Because beta blockers reduce both heart rate and blood pressure, in extreme circumstances lightheadedness and fainting may occur. These side effects are more likely in elderly patients, reinforcing the need for a cautious dosing approach.

Despite the potential side effects, beta blockers are a highly effective group of cardiac medications that provide overwhelming benefit with a low incidence of patient intolerance. For patients in whom beta blockers are proven to be beneficial, every effort should be made to include them as part of your regimen of prescription medication. Be sure to discuss this with your cardiologist.

ANGIOTENSIN CONVERTING ENZYME (ACE) INHIBITORS

ACE inhibitors primarily exert their benefits by directly lowering blood pressure. They do this by blocking a key hormonal pathway that is normally involved in constricting blood vessels.

ACE inhibitors are particularly helpful to patients with weakened heart muscle, including those who are suffering from congestive heart failure. Since ACE inhibitors lower blood pressure, they reduce the resistance to blood output and therefore the workload imposed upon the heart.

This favorable effect on heart workload is especially beneficial to patients with reduced heart-pumping function, as ACE inhibitors help stabilize the heart's pumping capacity and assist in reducing elevated heart pressures.

Also, after heart attack, ACE inhibitors can prevent adverse heart remodeling – an undesirable change in the geometry of the heart – and in so doing they reduce the possibility that a heart aneurysm will form.

When heart function is impaired, ACE inhibitors have been found to extend length of life and improve quality of life.

Based on well-conducted research, ACE inhibitors also appear to reduce heart attack and death rates in high-risk individuals, such as those with diabetes. How this occurs is unclear, but the benefit appears real.

In addition, ACE inhibitors help preserve kidney function in patients with diabetes.

In approximately 10 percent of patients taking ACE inhibitors, an annoying dry cough develops. This side effect can be reversed by either switching to another ACE inhibitor or switching to another medication in a closely related class. (See below, "Angiotensin Receptor Blockers.")

Hyperkalemia (elevated blood potassium) and kidney dysfunction may also occur but generally manifest in patients with preexisting kidney dysfunction or in patients with arterial blockages in the kidney (renal) arteries. This is not common, and if it occurs, it can be discovered and followed closely with simple blood tests.

ANGIOTENSIN RECEPTOR BLOCKERS

Angiotensin receptor blockers (ARBs) are typically given to patients who can't tolerate ACE inhibitors. As explained above, a minority of patients develops an ACE inhibitor-related cough.

As with beta blockers and ACE inhibitors, ARBs can help attenuate adverse ventricular remodeling – particularly in those patients who have suffered a recent heart attack – and also eventual weakening and dysfunction of the heart muscle.

ALDOSTERONE BLOCKERS

Aldosterone blockers are important in congestive heart failure when kidney blood flow may be reduced. By blocking the effects of the hormone aldosterone, which is inappropriately secreted during periods of reduced kidney blood flow, these medications help interrupt the cycle of sodium and fluid retention that is a dangerous part of congestive heart failure.

Potassium levels need to be monitored carefully in patients on aldosterone blockers, especially for those patients with kidney disease.

NITRATES

Nitrates dilate coronary arteries, peripheral arteries, and peripheral veins, thereby reducing blood pressure. The dilation gives prompt relief for symptoms of chest discomfort due to coronary artery blockages.

Nitrates are most well known in the form of nitroglycerin tablets or spray; typically, one tablet under the tongue or one quick spray will ameliorate symptoms. There are also extended- or delayed-release formulations in pill, patch, and paste formulations. Nitrates can improve the intensity and duration of symptom-free activity by reducing the frequency and severity of chest pain.

In patients with recurrent and predictable cardiac chest discomfort (stable angina pectoris), these formulations can be taken to preemptively reduce the frequency and severity of chest-pain episodes, especially when faced with a long walk or a tough journey up a steep hill or flight of stairs.

Nitrates are also available in an IV formulation. This is used in hospitalized patients with frequent and repetitive chest discomfort prior to a cardiac catheterization or before a strategy to increase blood flow has been determined.

As a class of medications, nitrates have not been found to reduce the incidence of heart attack or death rates that result. Instead, they have been found to reduce episodes of chest discomfort and – most important – to improve quality of life.

Because nitrates lower blood pressure they must be taken with caution. The immediate-release forms can lower blood pressure precipitously, so be sure to sit down when taking nitroglycerin under the tongue or in spray form. This way, if your blood pressure suddenly drops, you won't fall.

Do NOT take nitrates with ANY medications for erectile dysfunction. These two classes of medication can dangerously reduce blood pressure and can cause death. This is extremely important! If this is an issue for you, be sure to discuss it with your physician.

Do NOT take nitrates with ANY medications for erectile dysfunction. These two classes of medication can dangerously reduce blood pressure and can cause death. This is extremely important!

BLOOD-THINNERS

Aspirin is the most commonly prescribed cardiac medication. It is predominantly prescribed to patients with suspected or documented coronary artery disease, although it may also be used to prevent stroke in patients with atrial fibrillation or atrial flutter.

Aspirin inactivates blood platelets, the "sticky" components of the bloodstream that are needed for blood to clot. Because of its ability to stop blood platelets from sticking together, aspirin reduces the likelihood of blood-clot formation and therefore reduces the risk of stroke and heart attack. (Blood clots can form on unstable cholesterol plaques within the blood, causing near or total blockage of an artery, culminating in a stroke or heart attack.)

The equivalent of one-half of a full aspirin or two baby aspirins (162 mg daily) is believed to be the maximum daily dose necessary to render a positive effect on the heart.

In some patients, aspirin resistance has been discovered, whereby aspirin exerts a less-than-maximal effect on platelets. This possibility should be discussed with your physician as specific blood tests are available to test for resistance to aspirin.

If your doctor tells you to take aspirin, you should consider it an integral part of your treatment regimen and take it regularly. Since blood platelets possess an approximate seven-day lifespan, new blood platelets are continuously produced by the bone marrow, requiring a daily aspirin dose to render the newly made platelets inactive.

Side effects from daily aspirin intake can include easy bruising. Some patients may experience bleeding, as in nosebleeds or, more seriously, from the gastrointestinal tract. Bleeding episodes are infrequent and, unless you have a history of serious bleeding or a true aspirin allergy, there is no reason for you not to take aspirin. It should be prescribed to *all* people with coronary artery disease.

Thienopyridines, like aspirin, possess anti-platelet activity, but unlike the inactivating property of aspirin, thienopyridines interfere with molecules called receptors on the surface of platelet cells. Thienopyridines effectively block the receptors on the cell surface, preventing the platelets from adhering to one another and forming a blood clot.

This is different from the way aspirin works. Aspirin renders platelets inactive by irreversibly inactivating an important enzyme, cyclooxygenase. When thienopyridines are used *with* aspirin, a powerful dual anti-platelet effect ensues.

The most commonly prescribed member of this class of drugs is clopidogrel (better known by its brand name, Plavix).

As opposed to aspirin, this class of medications has not been proven to reduce the incidence of death or heart attacks. Thus, taking a thienopyridine is not indicated for patients with obstructive coronary artery disease that is stable (no intensifying symptoms). However, thienopyridines may be used in patients with stable coronary disease who have a serious, documented allergy or proven resistance to aspirin.

The benefits of thienopyridines are demonstrated in those patients who have had a coronary stent implanted. (A stent is like a miniature steel scaffold that holds open a coronary artery after it has been cleared of blockage.) Stent thrombosis (blood clot formation within a stent) is of particular concern with stents, especially those stents that are drug-coated. Thienopyridines markedly reduce the incidence of stent thrombosis.

Warfarin is an anticoagulant that exerts its effect by interfering with the hepatic (liver) synthesis of vitamin K-dependent clotting factors. This mechanism of action disrupts the blood-clotting cascade, thinning the blood and reducing the likelihood of clot formation.

Warfarin is most often prescribed for patients with intermittent and persistent atrial arrhythmias, such as atrial flutter and fibrillation; mechanical heart valves; or a severe restriction of mitral valve leaflet opening (termed mitral stenosis). In these circumstances, warfarin demonstrably reduces the risk of stroke.

Warfarin was one of the medications Dr. Smith prescribed for Robert's atrial flutter.

ANTI-ARRHYTHMIC MEDICATIONS

As a class, anti-arrhythmic medications aim to restore and maintain a normal heart rhythm. They are usually taken orally, but many also are available in IV formulations for use in select hospitalized patients.

Anti-arrhythmic medications do not cure heart-rhythm disturbances. Instead, they "control" the rhythm disturbances either by making them less frequent or by slowing the rate of the arrhythmia with each occurrence, lessening the effect on pulse rate and blood pressure, and therefore better maintaining blood flow.

Anti-arrhythmics can be used in combination with implantable cardiac defibrillators to reduce the incidence of arrhythmias and subsequent device shocks.

Heart-rhythm medications have the potential of making a heart-rhythm disturbance *worse.* (This is called a "pro-arrhythmic event.") For this reason, if you are prescribed an anti-arrhythmic, you may be hospitalized for a few days to have your ECG closely observed for any serious changes in the heart intervals and for any exacerbation of your heart arrhythmia Fortunately, when pro-arrhythmias occur, more than 90 percent are evident while the patient is still hospitalized, within the first 42 to 78 hours after medication treatment has begun.

Amiodarone is the most effective anti-arrhythmic medication available by prescription. It is indicated for both supraventricular and ventricular arrhythmias. It rarely causes pro-arrhythmias and can be safely started outside the hospital.

Unfortunately, its effectiveness needs to be counterbalanced by its potential toxicities, which include thyroid gland dysfunction, liver dysfunction, eye deposits, extreme sensitivity to sunlight, a bluish tinge to the skin, and lung toxicity.

The lung toxicity is the most feared problem. Pulmonary fibrosis (scarring on the lungs) may occur and is directly related to the total dose of amiodarone administered over time.

All these side effects can be averted with close monitoring of thyroid and liver blood tests, sun precautions, periodic chest x-rays, and formal breathing tests (pulmonary function tests) to measure lung volumes and capacity.

Although these side effects are serious, amiodarone is an extremely beneficial medication in certain situations and a "best choice" for select patients with atrial and ventricular arrhythmias that do not respond to other heart-rhythm medications. As with all medications, the use of amiodarone necessitates a careful discussion with your physician to assess the benefits and risks in your individual case.

If you are taking warfarin and are subsequently prescribed amiodarone, it is important to recognize that amiodarone interferes with warfarin, augmenting its effect. In fact, patients who take these medications in combination may require only half the dose of warfarin. It's vital that you discuss this with your doctor. This is an example of a medication interaction.

Beta blockers are the safest heart-rhythm medications, but also the least potent.

By reducing the effect of circulating adrenaline on the heart muscle, beta blockers mitigate the possibility that pro-arrhythmias will develop. While beta blockers rarely convert an abnormal rhythm to a normal rhythm, they are quite effective at maintaining a normal rhythm.

(You may remember that Dr. Smith prescribed metoprolol for Robert to help his rhythm remain normal.)

Flecainide is an anti-arrhythmic medication used for treating supraventricular arrhythmias, including atrial flutter and atrial fibrillation. It is generally a safe medication best reserved for patients with normal heart function, meaning that they show no evidence of previous heart attack or known obstructive coronary artery disease.

Because flecainide can slow cardiac conduction (the rate at which the heart conducts electrical impulses), periodic monitoring of the patient's electrocardiogram is required. This is most often done on an outpatient basis.

Sotalol is an anti-arrhythmic medication that also possesses beta-blocking qualities. Used predominantly for supraventricular arrhythmias, it is also used for ventricular heart-rhythm disturbances. The most common side effect of sotalol is fatigue.

Sotalol can unpredictably prolong electrocardiogram intervals. For this reason, patients are hospitalized when sotalol is initiated, with continuous monitoring of the heart rhythm (telemetry recording) and intermittent monitoring by electrocardiogram. It is an effective medication for maintaining a normal heart rhythm.

LIPID-MODIFYING MEDICATIONS

This group of medications reduces harmful lipids – LDL cholesterol and blood fats, also known as triglycerides – and increases beneficial HDL cholesterol. There are several classes to consider.

Statins are also known as HMG-CoA reductase inhibitors. HMG-CoA reductase is an important enzyme within the liver that is critical to cholesterol synthesis (formation). Statins interfere with this enzyme and directly reduce cholesterol formation.

Statins work mainly to lower LDL (bad) cholesterol levels and have smaller effects on increasing HDL (good) cholesterol and reducing triglyceride levels.

Statins also reduce the incidence of heart attacks and death rates among patients at high risk for coronary artery disease and those with confirmed coronary artery obstructions. The exact mechanism of this beneficial effect is not known but is believed to be related to their plaque-stabilization properties. High-dose statins have also been demonstrated to regress atherosclerotic plaque.

A heart attack is most commonly the result of a cholesterol plaque transitioning from a stable to unstable composition. An unstable plaque is more apt to fissure and rupture, increasing the likelihood of blood-clot formation, blood-clot adherence, and abrupt closure of the artery.

Statins help transition unstable plaques to greater stability, and they assist in maintaining plaque stability over the long term.

Plaque stability is not currently measurable, but advanced imaging techniques are being studied with the hope that unstable plaques can be identified and treated, perhaps with more intensive statin therapy and even preemptive stenting, before they rupture and cause a heart attack.

Statin Side Effects

If you take a statin, you'll need to be monitored periodically through blood-testing to assess for side effects.

The most common side effect is aching muscles. A blood test can be done to check the level of a muscle enzyme called creatinine phosphokinase (CPK).

Patients with muscle ache accompanied by an elevated CPK value are considered to be suffering myositis, a direct inflammatory injury of the muscle cells. When myositis is present, it is best to stop the statin. Myositis occurs in only a small percentage of patients and is completely reversible after stopping the statin.

Patients with muscle aches without CPK elevation are experiencing myalgia. This is not a form of muscle injury and does not warrant discontinuing the statin unless the symptoms are intolerable.

Liver inflammation is an infrequent side effect of statin therapy and can also be easily measured by a blood test. Most often, a baseline liver-enzyme blood level is obtained when a patient is started on a statin, with repeat values obtained three and six months later. If stable and normal, these tests are then repeated every six months.

If the liver enzymes rise to greater than three times their baseline value, the statin should be stopped. This extent of enzyme elevation occurs in only a small percentage of patients and is, again, completely reversible.

As with beta blockers, the side effects of statin medications are far outweighed by their established benefit. Statin medications save lives and are currently underprescribed to the kinds of patients who have been proven to benefit. If you have coronary artery disease, are at high risk for it, or have any documented atherosclerosis in your body and you are not taking a statin, ask your doctor why.

> If you have coronary artery disease, are at high risk for it, or have any documented atherosclerosis in your body and you are not taking a statin, ask your doctor why.

The **fibrates,** another class of medications, are used to target elevated triglycerides and low HDL (good) cholesterol levels. Fibrates lower triglycerides by reducing the liver's production of very-low-density lipoprotein (VLDL). (The VLDL particle is the particle that transports triglycerides within the bloodstream.)

Two common fibrates are gemfibrozil and fenofibrate. Gemfibrozil has been shown in one study to decrease the risk of heart attacks.

Fibrates can be administered with statins, which is desirable in patients with elevated levels of both triglycerides and LDL cholesterol. However, this combination of medications can raise the risk of muscle and liver toxicity. Therefore symptoms should be closely monitored along with serum levels of muscle and liver enzymes.

Other possible side effects include gastrointestinal upset and cholesterol-laden gallstone development, particularly in those patients on long-term fibrate therapy.

Fibrates can also enhance the blood-thinning effect of warfarin. If you take both warfarin and a fibrate, make sure that your blood-clotting time is carefully monitored. Most patients in this situation need less warfarin to achieve its desired effect.

Nicotinic acid, also known as niacin, is a component of vitamin B3. It is currently the best available treatment for raising HDL (good) cholesterol levels.

It acts by blocking the liver uptake of a major component of HDL cholesterol. This leaves higher levels of circulating HDL in the blood, allowing for enhanced removal of cholesterol by the liver.

Niacin also possesses a modest LDL cholesterol- and triglyceride-lowering effect.

Niacin, which was initially studied in the 1970s, has been shown to reduce heart attack and mortality rates.

The use of niacin has been limited by bothersome flushing. Flushing associated with niacin has been mitigated somewhat by use of the newer, slow-release formulations.

Also, niacin can elevate blood-sugar levels, which warrants close monitoring, especially in diabetic patients.

The recently introduced **cholesterol-absorption inhibitors** are an additional class of anti-hyperlipidemic medications.

Ezetimibe is the medication currently available in this class. This medication is a potent inhibitor of intestinal cholesterol absorption and reduces the overall delivery of cholesterol to the liver. The liver responds by generating more LDL (bad) cholesterol receptors, resulting in the uptake of more circulating LDL cholesterol and a lowering of LDL blood levels.

Ezetimibe can be safely used with statins. Their mechanisms of action are different and therefore complement each other. There is no known increase in liver or muscle toxicity when ezetimibe is prescribed with statins.

Side effects may include gastrointestinal upset and fatigue.

DIURETICS

Diuretics promote fluid loss. By removing excess fluid from the body, they improve a patient's energy level and exercise capacity.

Fluid retention is a significant problem for patients with congestive heart failure, so diuretics are a mainstay of medical treatment for that condition. They are also an effective means of managing blood pressure.

Diuretics may cause unwanted low levels of potassium and magnesium, in which case a dose adjustment is required. Your physician can adjust your dose depending upon how well they are working.

Other potential side effects include dehydration and reduced kidney blood flow, rendering the kidneys dysfunctional. Diuretic-induced kidney dysfunction is generally a reversible process once the patient is rehydrated.

Overzealous use of diuretics can lower blood pressure, induce lightheadedness, and in rare situations, cause fainting.

CALCIUM CHANNEL BLOCKERS

Calcium channel blockers, also known as calcium blockers, lower both heart rate and blood pressure by preventing the entry of calcium into the muscle cells of the heart and arteries.

Normally, calcium entering these cells causes the heart to contract and arteries to narrow. By impeding calcium's entry, calcium channel blockers decrease the vigor of cardiac contraction and dilate the arteries, resulting in lower blood pressure.

Calcium channel blockers also slow electrical cardiac conduction, thereby lowering the resting heart rate and the heart rate attained with exertion. Calcium channel blockers are prescribed for patients with elevated blood pressure and for patients with chronic angina whose symptoms are not relieved despite the use of beta blockers and nitrates at maximal doses.

Side effects of calcium channel blockers may include fatigue, lightheadedness, and constipation.

DIGOXIN

Digoxin, which has been around since the 1700s, has been a mainstay in the treatment of congestive heart failure by increasing the pumping function (contractility) of heart muscle.

In a recent study, digoxin was found to reduce hospitalization rates but not necessarily to increase longevity or otherwise improve quality of life for people with congestive heart failure.

Digoxin is cleared (metabolized) by the kidneys. In those patients with congestive heart failure and coexistent kidney dysfunction, digoxin must be carefully administered and its levels must be carefully monitored because high levels of digoxin may lead to heart-rhythm disturbances. Therefore, in these fragile patients who are experiencing associated kidney dysfunction, the risks of digoxin may outweigh the benefits.

Digoxin can also slow the heart rate, especially in those patients suffering atrial arrhythmias. Recently, beta blockers have supplanted digoxin for this purpose.

MANAGING YOUR MEDICATIONS

If your cardiologist prescribes medication, it is important that you discuss the rationale for the prescription, the expected benefits, any possible side effects, and the dosing strength and frequency.

You should also clarify whether you can expect to take this medication for a short time or are facing a lifelong commitment.

If cost is a factor, be direct with your physician and ask whether less expensive, equally effective alternatives exist. Often they do.

Also, be certain not to share medications with family members or friends. Dosages may not be the same, and each medication has a shelf life after which it may lose its desired effectiveness. No matter how close you are to your family or friends, it is safest to keep your medications separate from theirs.

Work with your pharmacist so that you understand whether the medication is to be taken on an empty stomach, with food, or on a full stomach after eating. Some medications are not affected by food intake.

Consider making a table or grid for yourself, delineating the medication name, dose, and dose-timing, and including the relationship to food intake. The table might look something like the one on the next page.

Taking your medications should be part of your daily routine. Your cardiologist should work with you to develop a medication regimen that is sustainable over time.

CURRENT MEDICATIONS				
Name	Dose	Frequency	Dose Timing	Relation to Food
Atenolol	25 mg	1 twice/day	10 a.m., 10 p.m.	None
Famotidine	20 mg	1 @ bedtime	10 p.m.	None
Aspirin	325 mg	1 each a.m.	10 a.m.	After food
Simvastatin	20 mg	1 @ bedtime	10 p.m.	None

Most medications are now available in formulations that require dosing no more frequently than twice a day. I tell my patients to put their medication bottles next to their toothbrush. In this way, they won't forget to take their medicines when they brush their teeth in the morning and again at night.

Missing a dose of an important medication, such as one that lowers blood pressure, can result in dangerous consequences.

For instance, missing a dose or abruptly stopping a beta blocker can be especially dangerous. Let me explain.

When you are taking beta blockers, the body's response is something called an up-regulation of beta receptors, which means that beta receptors multiply. If you suddenly stop taking the beta blocker, the up-regulated beta receptors remain and are exposed to circulating adrenaline, which can lead to a heightened cardiac response to the adrenaline.

By virtue of the elevated heart rate (tachycardia), this scenario could provoke cardiac chest discomfort, exacerbate heart failure, and increase the likelihood of serious cardiac rhythm disturbances.

Abrupt cessation of diuretics can also be critical, as fluid may rapidly accumulate. Patients with heart failure may not have the cardiac muscle reserve to accommodate this increase in fluid and thus may get into trouble quickly. ◆

NEVER stop taking any cardiac medication suddenly. Doing so can have dangerous effects on your heart. Instead, consult with your doctor.

A Final Note

As you can see, preparing for a cardiology appointment and optimizing your relationship with your cardiologist are not last-minute endeavors.

They require both careful thought about why you are seeking help and an up-to-date inventory of your current symptoms.

Compiling your past medical and surgical histories and an accurate list of your present and past medications will also enhance your visit and relationship by facilitating a smooth exchange of information. I often tell my patients that a successful doctor-patient relationship is a 50-50 proposition. The patient's part is to prepare carefully for the appointment, keep the physician up-to-date on any symptom changes, and follow through on the physician's recommendations.

The doctor must contribute equally by being an excellent diagnostician and a skilled and respectful communicator.

If these criteria are met, the doctor-patient relationship is almost always a "win-win."

Appendix

PREPARING FOR A
DOCTOR'S APPOINTMENT

CHIEF COMPLAINT

What is the reason you are seeing the doctor?

HISTORY OF PRESENT ILLNESS

(E.g., discomfort in your chest. Elaborate on your chief complaint, including the duration, location, and character of the discomfort, the precipitating and alleviating factors, and what you were doing when the discomfort began.)

HISTORY

- Medical history (e.g., hypertension – 6 years, average blood pressure 120/80 on medications)
- Surgical history (e.g., appendectomy – 1972 – age 8 years, Jackson Hospital, Jackson, Michigan)

PRESENT MEDICATIONS

- E.g., Losartan for high blood pressure, 25 mg once per day – 3 years

PAST MEDICATIONS

- E.g., Lisinopril 5 mg once per day – 1 year, discontinued due to a cough side effect

ALLERGIES

- E.g., sulfa medications – severe rash

SOCIAL HISTORY

- Marital status
- Occupation
- Number of children

HABITS

- Tobacco (e.g., cigarettes – one pack per day from age 30 to 60, quit five years ago)
- Alcohol (e.g., none, past or present)
- Exercise (e.g., 30 minutes of treadmill work, three days per week)
- Diet (e.g., fast food three times per week)
- High-risk activities or hobbies (e.g., skydiving)

OBSTETRICS AND GYNECOLOGICAL HISTORY (IF APPLICABLE)

- Number of pregnancies
- Number of live births
- Gynecological surgery history (can also be located in the past surgery section)

PREVENTIVE MEDICINE STATUS

- Immunizations (e.g., tetanus vaccine, 2002)
- Last eye examination and findings
- Last Pap test and results (if applicable)
- Last mammogram and results (if applicable)
- Last colonoscopy and results
- Last prostate exam and PSA blood-test results (if applicable)

FAMILY HISTORY

- E.g., father deceased, age 62
  (hypertension, heart attack, stroke)

REVIEW OF SYSTEMS

A general review of each body system and a list of associated
symptoms/concerns

- E.g., head – headaches for four years, now more frequent
  and intense, lasting for 15 to 30 minutes

- E.g., eyes – excessive watering during April and May,
  reading vision not as clear

- E.g., lungs – wheezing noticeable during heavy exertion,
  occasional nonproductive cough

MISCELLANEOUS QUESTIONS AND CONCERNS

A good place to organize your questions and concerns before
your appointment

- E.g. – I have been more short of breath recently and have
  noticed wheezing. Are these symptoms something I should
  be concerned about?

Index

hyperlipidemia, 78, 108-110, 150-153

hypertension, 110-113
  ambulatory monitoring, 62-63
  aneurysms and, 78-79
  arrhythmias, 50, 93, 126, 136-137
  medications, 111, 141, 143-144, 153, 154
  pulmonary, 103

hypertensive heart disease, 136-137

hypertrophic cardiomyopathy, 50-51, 113-114

I

imaging
  cardiac catheterization (coronary angiogram), 8, 25, 67-70
  cardiac CT, 70-71
  cardiac MRI, 72-73
  carotid vascular ultrasound, 99
  computed tomography angiogram (CT angio/CTA), 71-72
  Doppler color-flow, 64
  echocardiogram, 15, 50, 63-65, 82, 84, 92
  nuclear imaging, 65-66
  transesophageal echocardiography (TEE), 82, 84, 92

immune system, 58

implantable cardiac defibrillator (ICD), 133-134

Internet, information, 48, 142
  See also websites

interventional cardiology, 15

intracoronary stent, 69

invasive cardiologist, 67

ischemia, 41

K

kidney function, 113, 144, 145, 154

L

LDL cholesterol, 108-110, 150-153

left ventricular hypertrophy, 85

legs
  atherosclerosis in, 101-102, 128

lipids
  hyperlipidemia, 78, 108-110
  medications for, 150-153

liver inflammation, 151-152

loop recorders, 74-75

lungs, 57, 86, 93, 103, 149

lymphatic system, 58

M

magnesium, 153

mantle radiation, 38

Marfan's syndrome, 79

mediastinum, 127

medical history, 6-7, 37-40
  family history, 49-52

medical records
  electronic, 56-57
  organizing, 38-40

medications
  abbreviations on, 43
  ACE inhibitors, 111, 125, 143-144
  aldosterone blockers, 145
  allergies, 46, 49, 58, 147
  angiotensin receptor blockers (ARBs), 144
  anti-arrhythmic, 148-150
  antiplatelet, 122
  aspirin, 124-125, 146, 147
  beta blockers, 111, 125, 131, 136, 141, 143, 149-150, 156
  blood-thinners, 122, 146-148, 152
  calcium channel blockers, 154
  cholesterol-lowering, 109, 150-153
  clot-busters, 121, 122-123
  digoxin, 154-155
  diuretics, 153-154, 156
  erectile dysfunction, 146
  fibrates, 152
  herbal preparations, 45

OTHER BOOKS FROM
CLEVELAND CLINIC PRESS

Age Well! A Cleveland Clinic Guide

Arthritis: A Cleveland Clinic Guide

Autopsy – Learning from the Dead: A Cleveland Clinic Guide

Battling the Beast Within: Success in Living with Adversity
(about multiple sclerosis)

Breastless in the City: A Young Woman's Story of Love, Loss,
and Breast Cancer

Epilepsy – Information for You and Those Who Care About You:
A Cleveland Clinic Guide

Forever Home
(a chapter book for young readers)

Getting a Good Night's Sleep: A Cleveland Clinic Guide

The Granny-Nanny: A Guide for Parents and Grandparents
Who Share Child Care

Headaches: A Cleveland Clinic Handbook

Heart Attack: A Cleveland Clinic Guide

Heroes with a Thousand Faces: True Stories of People with Facial
Deformities and Their Quest for Acceptance

Lessons Learned: Stroke Recovery from a Caregiver's Perspective

My Grampy Can't Walk
   (a children's picture book about multiple sclerosis)

One Stroke, Two Survivors
   (the journey of a stroke victim and his wife)

Overcoming Infertility: A Cleveland Clinic Guide

Planting the Roses: A Cancer Survivor's Story
   (about esophageal cancer)

Sober Celebrations: Lively Entertaining Without the Spirits
   (alcohol-free cooking)

Stop Smoking Now! The Rewarding Journey to a Smoke-Free Life

Tango: Lessons for Life
   (a dancing doctor's perspective on healing and life)

Thyroid Disorders: A Cleveland Clinic Guide

To Act As A Unit: The Story of the Cleveland Clinic
   (fourth edition)

Women's Health – Your Body, Your Hormones, Your Choices:
   A Cleveland Clinic Guide

Write for Life: Healing Body, Mind, and Spirit Through
   Journal Writing

You CAN Eat That! Awesome Food for Kids with Diabetes

CLEVELAND CLINIC PRESS

Cleveland Clinic Press publishes nonfiction trade books for the medical, health, nutrition, cookbook, and children's markets. It is the mission of the Press to increase the health literacy of the American public and to dispel myths and misinformation about medicine, health care, and treatment. Our authors include leading authorities from Cleveland Clinic as well as a diverse list of experts drawn from medical and health institutions whose research and treatment breakthroughs have helped countless people.

Each Cleveland Clinic Guide provides the health-care consumer with practical and authoritative information. Every book is reviewed for accuracy and timeliness by Cleveland Clinic experts.

www.clevelandclinicpress.org

CLEVELAND CLINIC

Cleveland Clinic, located in Cleveland, Ohio, is a not-for-profit multispecialty academic medical center that integrates clinical and hospital care with research and education. Cleveland Clinic was founded in 1921 by four renowned physicians with a vision of providing outstanding patient care based upon the principles of cooperation, compassion, and innovation. *U.S. News & World Report* consistently names Cleveland Clinic as one of the nation's best hospitals in its annual "America's Best Hospitals" survey. Approximately 1,500 full-time salaried physicians at Cleveland Clinic and Cleveland Clinic Florida represent more than 120 medical specialties and subspecialties. In 2006, patients came for treatment from every state and 100 countries.

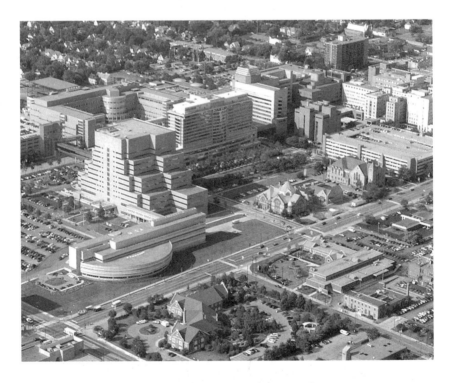

www.clevelandclinic.org